Discovering the Human Connectome

Discovering the Human Connectome

Olaf Sporns

The MIT Press
Cambridge, Massachusetts
London, England

MIT Press books may be purchased at special quantity discounts for business or sales promotional use. For information, please email special_sales@mitpress.mit.edu or write to Special Sales Department, The MIT Press, 55 Hayward Street, Cambridge, MA 02142.

This book was set in Syntax and Times Roman by Toppan Best-set Premedia Limited. Printed and bound in the United States of America.

Library of Congress Cataloging-in-Publication Data

Sprons, Olaf.
Discovering the human connectome / Olaf Sporns.
   p. ;   cm.
Includes bibliographical references and index.
ISBN 978-0-262-01790-9 (hardcover : alk. paper)
I. Title.
[DNLM: 1. Brain—anatomy & histology. 2. Brian—physiology. 3. Brain Mapping. 4. Models, Neurological. WL 300]
612.8'2—dc23
2012006719

10 9 8 7 6 5 4 3 2 1

For Anita

Contents

Preface

In the early summer of 2005 my colleagues Rolf Kötter, Giulio Tononi, and I put the finishing touches to a review article (really a position paper) somewhat ambitiously entitled "The Human Connectome: A Structural Description of the Human Brain" (Sporns et al., 2005). At the time, the connectome was just an idea, nothing more. The idea seemed simple enough. The human brain is a complex network whose operation depends on how its neurons are linked to each other. When attempting to understand the workings of a complex network, one must know how its elements are connected, and how these elements and connections cooperate to generate network function. The human connectome describes the complete set of all neural connections of the human brain. It thus constitutes a network map that is of fundamental importance for studies of brain dynamics and function. When I googled the term "connectome" (just to be sure no one else had thought of it earlier) I remember getting around 10 hits, none of them relevant to the brain. In fact, some of them were oddly irrelevant—I recall finding "connect-to-me" (a dating site, I believe) and "connect-home" among the search results. As of April 2012 the same Google search returns nearly a quarter million hits. What happened?

The simple idea of mapping the connections of the human brain in their entirety has captured the imagination of many, not only neuroscientists but also researchers in adjoining fields interested in human cognition, brain and mental disorders, and complex systems and networks, as well as members of the general public. I believe it is fair to say that the connectome and the nascent field of connectomics are beginning to influence the ways many neuroscientists collect, analyze, and think about their data. Connectomics is directed at integrative function—central to connectomics is the notion that the brain can be described and understood as a *network*, not just by way of a metaphor but in the precise technical and mathematical sense of a connectivity graph. Adopting this view opens new horizons on brain function, and it allows the use of powerful analytic tools and concepts coming from the emerging science of complex networks. In my previous book *Networks of the Brain*, I made the case that neuroscience has much to gain from adopting this theoretical framework, and I attempted to sketch a first draft of an integrative theory of brain function that is based on network architectures and mechanisms. The present book builds on this theoretical framework to ask some very specific questions. What is the nature of the human connectome? Why is it important to pursue the connectome as a high-priority scientific goal, and what will the connectome tell us once we have discovered it? What are the most compelling empirical strategies for mapping the human connectome, and how can we make sense of the extraordinary amount of data they will deliver? What is the future promise and, equally importantly, what are the limitations of connectomics in neuroscience?

Today, the human connectome is known to us only in broad outline, and intensive research under way in many laboratories and research centers around the world will add substantially to our understanding of human brain connectivity over coming years. While future iterations of this book will undoubtedly deliver a much more refined and detailed picture of the connectome, some of the basic concepts and theoretical ideas that lie at the origin of connectomics will likely remain valid. Central among these ideas is the notion that the connectome is a complex network and that a detailed account of network structure and function can deliver a much needed new perspective on brain function. One of the biggest challenges will be to discover how these networks shape the integrated and dynamic activity of neurons and brain regions and how the network architecture of our brain relates to our behavioral and cognitive capacities. I suspect that meeting this challenge will take far longer than attaining the first goal of creating an accurate and detailed map of human brain connectivity. Connectomics as a comprehensive research effort directed at understanding the brain as a complex network will occupy us for some time to come. We are only at the very beginning of what promises to be an exciting new period of empirical investigation and theoretical inquiry.

The connectome might never have become a reality, at least not with a prominent focus on the human brain, without my longtime colleague and friend Rolf Kötter. Rolf and I first talked about a future project to map all of the connections of the human brain in November 2004 at a meeting near Toronto, organized by Randy McIntosh and sponsored by the J.S. McDonnell Foundation. We continued to pursue our discussion via frequent e-mail and phone conversations and started to generate a draft of a "white paper" outlining a detailed proposal for mapping the human connectome. I fondly remember a long discussion on a cold morning in early March 2005, over breakfast in a café outside the National Science Foundation in Arlington (we were both members of a review panel). We had already sketched out the main rationale for the connectome, and we were pondering how we might gain broader support and acceptance for the concept in our field (perhaps even from funding agencies!). Both of us were unsure about the project's feasibility in the near term, but we convinced each other that, despite these uncertainties, it was important to make a public argument that laid out the motivation for the connectome as a foundational network model of the brain. We formulated a multistep plan for the project, including diffusion and functional magnetic resonance imaging as well as electromagnetic recordings across a large population to assess individual variability. Within a few weeks the article was written and submitted, and eventually published in the journal *PLoS Computational Biology*. Over the years, the idea of the connectome gathered momentum, driven by new techniques and the discoveries of many colleagues in the field. Rolf and I were tremendously excited when, in 2009, the Human Connectome Project finally moved forward under National Institutes of Health (NIH) sponsorship, something neither of us had envisioned even a few years earlier. I am deeply saddened that Rolf will not be with us on the journey toward discovering the human connectome. His untimely death after a long battle with a devastating disease was a profound and tragic loss to our research community. Rolf's vision and insight, his scholarly wisdom, and his warm collegiality (and dry sense of humor) will be missed dearly.

My own research described in this book has been generously sponsored by the J.S. McDonnell Foundation and, more recently, by the NIH under the auspices of the Human Connectome Project. I wrote the book with the support of a 2011 John Simon Guggenheim Memorial Fellowship and while on sabbatical leave at Indiana University. I owe thanks to many colleagues for the inspiration their work has given me. It is an extraordinary privilege to be one among many investigators collaborating on the NIH's Human Connectome Project, under the leadership of David Van Essen and Kamil Ugurbil. I have no doubt that the project will be a major milestone on the road toward understanding the workings of the human brain. While the ideas laid out in this book are entirely my own, I do hope that some of them will be of use in ongoing and future connectome projects.

Many colleagues have encouraged me to write this book, and I thank them for their support and intellectual generosity in sharing ideas and opinions. Mika Rubinov graciously volunteered to read draft chapters, and his input has been extremely useful. I am grateful to Michael Breakspear, Kevin Briggman, Yoonsuck Choe, Patric Hagmann, Martijn van den Heuvel, Marc Joliot, Christoph Palm, Marc Raichle, and David Van Essen for generously providing figures and other materials. I thank Bob Prior at MIT Press for allowing me to become (in his words) a "repeat offender" by supporting my second book project in three years. Finally, I thank my wife, Anne Prieto, for her love and support—and I promise I won't do this again so soon!

1 Introduction

If I had to point to the single most important thing to know about how the brain works, my answer would be "connectivity." Of course, much else comes to mind—the interplay of ionic currents that generate neuronal membrane potentials, the variety of neurotransmitter systems involved in synaptic transmission and plasticity, the capacity of neurons to convert inputs into outputs, the endlessly rich patterns of cellular and synaptic morphology, and many other features of the brain at molecular, cellular, and systems scales. And yet, I believe it is fair to say that the brain's computational power depends critically (though certainly not entirely) on how individual processing elements are networked together. The human brain is a network of extraordinary complexity, an intricate web of billions of neurons connected by trillions of synapses and wiring that spans a distance halfway to the moon. How this network is connected is important for virtually all facets of the brain's integrative function (Sporns, 2011a). Brain connectivity allows neurons to exhibit an extraordinary range of physiological responses and enables them to generate and distribute information, to coordinate their activity over short and long distances, and to retain a structural record of past events.

The centerpiece of brain connectivity is the connectome—a comprehensive description of how neurons and brain regions are interconnected. Much of this book is about current efforts to chart these connections in the human brain and what the first maps created with a variety of techniques tell us about the brain's network architecture. To be sure, the insights we have gained so far are preliminary and incomplete, and there is much still to be discovered. However, the journey toward mapping the human connectome has begun, and significant progress is being made at an ever-accelerating pace. A growing number of empirical and theoretical studies of the brain's network architecture and dynamics are laying the groundwork for the nascent field of connectomics. The main goal of this book is to describe the origins and prospects of the endeavor and to chart its main scientific and intellectual underpinnings.

The book is arranged in eight chapters. This first chapter positions the connectome within the wider context of biological systems by examining the role of structure for understanding biological function, the nature of complexity, and the importance of networks in making sense of brain connectivity. It also provides an introduction to basic concepts and terminology of graphs and network models. Chapter 2 offers a more detailed treatment of the conceptual foundations of the connectome, and chapter 3 focuses on some of the challenges posed by the connectome's multiscale architecture, the inherent variability of nervous systems, and the ongoing structural change that continually remodels neurons and connections. Chapters 4 and 5 survey current empirical strategies for mapping the connectome, covering the entire range of approaches from electron microscopy to magnetic resonance imaging (MRI). I will explore the merits of each technology and ask how these approaches may be integrated to yield a coherent map linking cellular connectivity to brain systems. Chapter 6 deals with how the connectome generates temporal structure in neuronal dynamics. I will also reflect on the important role of "functional connectomics" for linking brain networks to human behavior. Chapters 7 and 8 cover the significant impact of connectomics on computational studies of the nervous system, including the emerging picture of network organization delivered by graph analysis, the need for advanced neuroinformatics tools, and the progress made toward building comprehensive computational models of the human brain. I end by attempting to forecast some of the innovations that connectomics will bring to both basic and translational neuroscience.

Before squarely focusing on the brain, let us briefly look at how the notion of the connectome as a structural foundation for understanding brain function fits with related and more general ideas about the role of structure in the biological sciences. Two ideas are central to the endeavor, the importance of structure for shaping biological function and the role of networks for coordinating the actions of components into coherent system dynamics.

Structure and Complexity

The importance of structure for the functioning of biological systems can hardly be overstated. Examples are found everywhere, ranging from macromolecules to whole organisms. Structure strongly determines the physicochemical attributes of biomolecules, including their locations within the cell and their interactions with other molecular species. The iconic double-helix structure of deoxyribonucleic acid (DNA), widely considered one of the most important scientific discoveries of the 20th century, "immediately suggests a possible copying mechanism for the genetic material" (Watson and Crick, 1953, p. 737). The chemical specificity of enzymes is largely determined by their shape and geometry, which permit interactions with substrates, inhibitors, and activators. Virtually all electrical properties of neuronal membranes depend on the actions of transmembrane protein channels that regulate the passage of specific ions across the cell surface (figure 1.1). Their stable placement within the membrane, the aggregation of protein subunits to form a nanometer scale pore, the selectivity of the channel for specific ions, and the gating of channels in response to chemical ligands or changes in the cell's

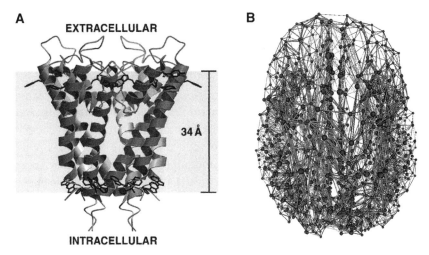

Figure 1.1
The importance of structure in biological function. (A) Schematic representation of the protein structure of the potassium channel. The diagram shows the folding pattern of the four channel subunits and its integration into the cell membrane, here shaded in gray. The channel forms a pore through which potassium ions can cross. Its structure enables the fundamental biological process of selective membrane conductance which underlies all electrical signaling among neurons. The image is reproduced with permission from Doyle et al. (1998). (B) Schematic representation of the network of fiber tracts coursing through the human brain's white matter. The nodes correspond to a set of cortical regions covering both cerebral hemispheres, and the edges between them correspond to neural connections. The structure of this network shapes neural activity across the brain and forms the anatomical basis of large-scale brain function. The image was kindly provided by Martijn van den Heuvel (University Medical Center Utrecht, The Netherlands).

membrane potential all depend on the spatial configuration of the channel's molecular components.

Relations between structure and function are also evident at larger scales, in the shape and form of organelles, cells, tissues, organs, and even in the biomechanics of the whole organism. An organism's behavioral repertoire is shaped by numerous structural and mechanical constraints, from the basic layout of the body's sensors and effectors to the articulation of limbs or wings and the couplings of muscles and connective tissues. As a whole, the anatomical organization of the musculoskeletal system supports the stability and adaptive control of bodily motion and behavior. The importance of structure and biological form extends to the nervous system, and how this structural organization shapes brain function is the central theme of this book. The brain's numerous anatomical components and their physical couplings are critically important for its functional activity, the flow of neural signals that underlies all mental experience. Structural linkages between elements of neuronal systems channel their dynamic interactions and constrain the paths across which neurons can communicate and share information (see figure 1.1). Just as the network of chemical bonds comprising a macromolecule determines which of its subdomains fold into spatial proximity,[1] the brain's network of synaptic connections determines the similarity and specificity of functional and physiological attributes among neuronal collectives.

The importance of structure does not imply that structure alone can fully predict all functional outcomes or that full knowledge of structure allows a keen observer to deduce all of the physiology and behavior of a biological system. For function to be properly expressed, structure has to be placed into a wider context. In the case of biomolecules, this context is supplied by the roughly 10^{12} molecules making up a cell—a function of a protein channel such as voltage-gating, while certainly dependent on its molecular configuration, requires a surrounding neuron and its membrane potential. In the case of the brain, context comes from internal as well as sensory signals, for example those caused by the behaviors of a social group—neuronal activity related to emotional constructs such as empathy, while caused by connectivity in the brain, also reflects interpersonal processes occurring in a social environment.

In addition to context, structure and function must also be viewed as engaging in a continuous dialogue. Just as structure shapes function, the emergence of new functions often depends on making structural changes. Heritable modification of the structural arrangement of molecules, cells, or tissues is one way by which selectional forces operating on an evolutionary time scale can mold biological function. Selection based on function is ultimately responsible for the kinds of structures we find as part of organisms today. In the case of the brain, alterations in neural circuitry contribute to the emergence of new behaviors or cognitive capacities. Function itself leaves a structural record as is amply demonstrated by the many structural traces left as a result of neuronal activity.

This consideration of the centrality of structure–function relationships leads us to two important aspects shared by most, if not all, biological systems. They are *multiscale systems* that are organized as *complex networks*. Biological processes unfold on multiple scales that range from molecules to organisms and span 10 and 15 orders of magnitude in space and time, respectively (e.g., Hunter and Borg, 2003; figure 1.2). Importantly, these scales interact and are mutually interdependent. No scale is privileged over others in the sense that system behavior cannot be fully reduced to processes occurring at one scale only. At each scale, and across scales, biological systems are organized as networks, consisting of a large number of components that are connected in complex patterns. It is the coordinated action of networks that is responsible for global functional properties of cells and organisms.

Understanding the global functional properties of a biological system requires knowledge about the system's elements as well as a map of how these elements mutually interact. Significant research efforts in areas such as ecology and biodiversity, cancer biology, cellular signal transduction, metabolism and gene regulation, and, finally, neuroscience are directed toward mapping the structure of complex biological networks. As it turns out, the research program of connectomics closely parallels that of the relatively new field of "systems biology."

Connectomics and Systems Biology

A major aim of systems biology is the application of mathematical and computational models in areas such as population biology, enzyme kinetics, biochemical pathways, and genetic regulatory circuits. The inception of systems biology coincided with the arrival of large-scale genomics and proteomics data sets (Ideker et al., 2001; Kitano, 2001).[2] These data sets required concerted efforts to collect, store, visualize, and integrate large amounts of biological information. Building on data about genes and proteins, the overarching goal of systems biology is to account for the molecular origins of emergent biological phenomena: "Systems biology is a scientific discipline that endeavors to quantify all of the molecular

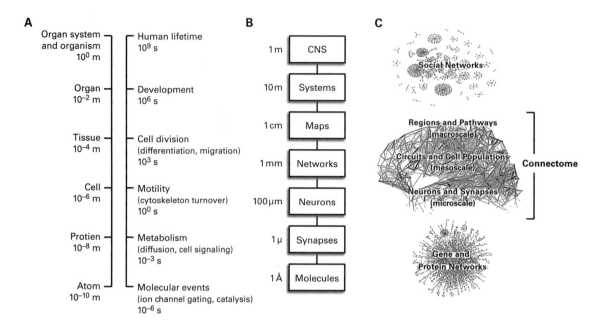

Figure 1.2
Levels of organization in biological systems and in the brain. (A) Spatial and temporal scales, spanning many orders of magnitudes. Similar diagrams can be found in Hunter and Borg (2003) and Dada and Mendes (2011). (B) Levels of organization in the nervous system. The diagram is adapted from a similar illustration in Churchland and Sejnowski (1992). CNS, central nervous system. (C) The nervous system as a hierarchy of networks. The multiscale networks of the connectome are interspersed between networks operating at cellular and social scales.

elements of a biological system to assess their interactions and to integrate that information into graphical network models that serve as predictive hypotheses to explain emergent behaviors" (Hood et al., 2004, p. 640). Hiroaki Kitano poignantly expressed the principal aim of systems biology as going beyond static descriptions of the inventory of genes and proteins. A biological system, in his words, "is not just an assembly of genes and proteins, [and] its properties cannot be fully understood merely by drawing diagrams of interconnections. Although such a diagram represents an important first step, it is analogous to a static roadmap, whereas what we really seek to know are the traffic patterns, why such traffic patterns emerge, and how we can control them" (Kitano, 2002, p. 1662).

Several aspects of systems biology set it apart from more traditional research approaches (Aitchison and Galitski, 2003). In addition to "hypothesis-driven" investigation, systems biology includes an important component of "discovery science." Discovery science involves the analysis of large data sets with the explicit goals of identifying significant statistical patterns, which can then lead to the formulation of new hypotheses. By charting the elementary components of functional systems and their dynamic interactions, systems biology aims at discovering the network architecture of biological systems. To accomplish this aim and to effectively bridge system structure and function, systems biology must integrate data from disparate sources and across levels of organization. Finally, the overall research effort is directed at creating plausible models of biological systems that can be tested, as hypotheses, against empirical data (figure 1.3). These models are formulated within a quantitative mathematical modeling framework and allow researchers to examine the dependency of global state transitions on specific system variables or to predict global system responses to specific perturbations.

Systems biology draws on the creation of large-scale data sets that record comprehensive information about specific domains of biology and that lay the material foundations for entire subdisciplines. These data sets are often labeled with the suffix "ome," signifying that they comprise a complete set of elementary components within their respective domain of knowledge. The first was the genome, a term coined in 1920 by the geneticist Hans Winkler.[3] Other "omes" that have proven useful in molecular and cellular biology include the proteome (the complete set of proteins expressed by a specific cell or organism), the transcriptome (the set of RNA molecules), the metabolome (the set of metabolites), and the interactome (the set of molecular interactions, for example, between proteins, in a specific cell or organism).[4] Some "omes" primarily record molecular components while others (like the interactome) explicitly refer to networks of interactions (Giot et al., 2003; Li et al., 2004). While not all "omes," once coined, turn out to be viable additions to the biological repertoire, several "omes" such as the genome and interactome have unquestionable utility that derives from their universality (they apply to all living forms), their totality (each comprises a complete set of data), and their permanence (the genome of an organism, once determined, does not change with time).[5]

Beyond semantic similarities, there are several reasons why the connectome belongs in the family of complex biological systems and why connectomics represents an extension of systems biology into the realm of neuroscience.[6] Mirroring the approach of systems biology, connectomics draws on cumulative and foundational data about components and interactions. The connectome records structure in all organisms with a nervous system (universality), comprises a complete description of

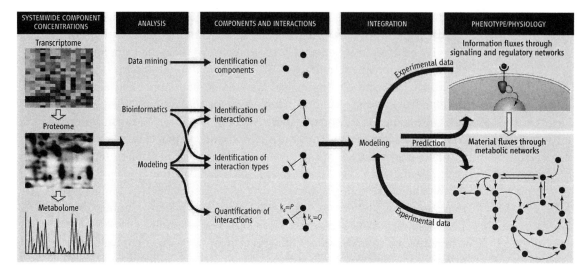

Figure 1.3
Models in systems biology. This schematic diagram illustrates the major data and modeling components of systems biology and how they relate to each other. On the left are comprehensive system-wide measurements of transcripts, proteins, and metabolites. Data analysis efforts identify system components and interactions, which feed into explicit computational models that lead to predictions of new data. Models are continually refined by feedback from experiments. Modified (converted to grayscale) and reproduced with permission from Sauer et al. (2007).

brain connectivity (totality), and, once determined, serves as a lasting resource and foundation for future research (permanence). Like systems biology, connectomics goes beyond static "wiring diagrams" to account for the rich dynamics that emerge from complex brain networks. The connectome's primary goal is the collection of information on structural brain networks comprised of neurons and synapses; however, the wider aim of connectomics includes an account of how this static network is transcribed into dynamic brain activity and behavior. Connectomics is a cumulative scientific effort, involving the collection of very large data sets on brain connectivity that are shared and made available across a broad research community. Finally, connectomics has a strong discovery-science component, and it relies on statistical and computational models for the interpretation and analysis of large data sets in order to generate new questions and hypotheses about brain function.[7]

The "omics" revolution, as it is sometimes called, brings with it the formidable challenge of representing and integrating large-scale foundational data sets to allow their interpretation in the context of the workings of the cell or organism (Joyce and Palsson, 2007). Computation and modeling play an important part in meeting this challenge, and as a result the fields of bioinformatics and computational biology have experienced significant growth over recent years. Both fields have profited from the development of new modeling techniques and approaches. Computational models of biological systems need to capture phenomena on different temporal and spatial scales and thus require integration of physical and biological processes across different levels of organization (Coveney and Fowler, 2005; Southern et al., 2008; Dada and Mendes, 2011). In some areas of computational biology, multiscale models are by now quite well developed. For example, multiscale models of organ systems such as the human heart have successfully integrated information across micro- and macroscales (Noble, 2002). Based on an anatomically detailed structural description of the heart, these models simulate its mechanical and electrical dynamics. Components at the microscale include membrane currents and ion pumps to model voltage changes across cardiac muscle cell membranes, resulting in waves of excitation unfolding across the tissue. Models of current flow and muscle cell contraction are combined to create a description of the deformation dynamics of the myocardium through the cardiac cycle. The result is an integrative account of electrical activation, pulsation, and blood flow at the macroscale, based on microscale mechanisms simulated in conjunction with a structural model of heart tissue.

An important conceptual foundation for thinking about complex biological systems comes from the science of networks. Cataloguing system components and their relations is only a first step toward the ambitious goal of understanding how their dynamic interactions give rise to integrated functional states. Network analysis and modeling offers an attractive and by now widely adopted theoretical framework for translating components and relations into global system behavior. A full exploration of the many applications of network approaches in neuroscience is beyond the scope of this book (instead, see Sporns, 2011a). However, a brief survey of network methodology and terminology is needed to set the stage for much of what is to come. Let us turn to an overview of how brain networks can be described and analyzed with modern quantitative approaches.

Networks of the Brain

Network diagrams are ubiquitous in the neurobiological literature and have long served as useful devices to summarize anatomical and physiological relationships among circuit elements (figure 1.4). The discovery of the cellular architecture of the brain in the 19th century first revealed the nervous system as a complex aggregate of seemingly innumerable nerve cells interconnected in ways that were anatomically organized and specific to each part of the brain. The "neuron theory" motivated early theoretical accounts directed at linking psychological phenomena to their anatomical and physiological substrates. Examples are Theodor Meynert's attempts at deciphering brain architectures (see chapter 5), Sigmund Freud's anticipation of changes in neuronal connections as the material basis of memory in his (then unpublished) 1895 manuscript entitled *A Project for a Scientific Psychology* (Freud, 1966), and Sigmund Exner's early network diagrams. In the opening passage of his treatise *Entwurf zu einer Physiologischen Erklärung der Psychischen Erscheinungen*, Exner expressed his central goal "to trace the most prominent psychological phenomena back to differential excitation of nerves and nerve centers, that is, to link the diversity of consciousness to quantitative relations and differences in the central connections of otherwise equivalent nerves and centers" (Exner, 1894, p. 3).[8]

However, the quantitative framework for describing those differences in connections of "nerves and centers" was missing. While the origins of graph theory extend back over 250 years, its prominence as a model for complex social and biological systems composed of numerous elements and interactions is a fairly recent phenomenon. Beginning in the 1930s with "sociograms," graphical descriptions of interpersonal relationships between members of a social group, the full power of network analysis as a quantitative model for sociological theory was realized only much later. In a seminal paper written almost 40 years ago, the sociologist Mark Granovetter proposed that network theory could address what he saw as the fundamental weakness in his field, "that it does not relate micro-level interactions to macro-level patterns in any convincing way" (Granovetter, 1973, p. 1360). He went on to suggest that "it is through [...] networks that small-scale interaction becomes translated into large-scale patterns, and that these, in turn, feed back into small groups."[9] Network theory has since undergone enormous expansion in virtually all areas of the social and natural sciences. Most recently, it has become an integral part of sophisticated analysis and modeling of biological systems at cellular and organismic scales (Barabási and Oltvai, 2004; Zhu et al., 2007; Bascompte, 2007).

Networks or graphs are collections of nodes and edges, with edges representing relationships between pairs of nodes. In the case of the

A   B

C   L1

L2

L3

P

I

100μm

000329C

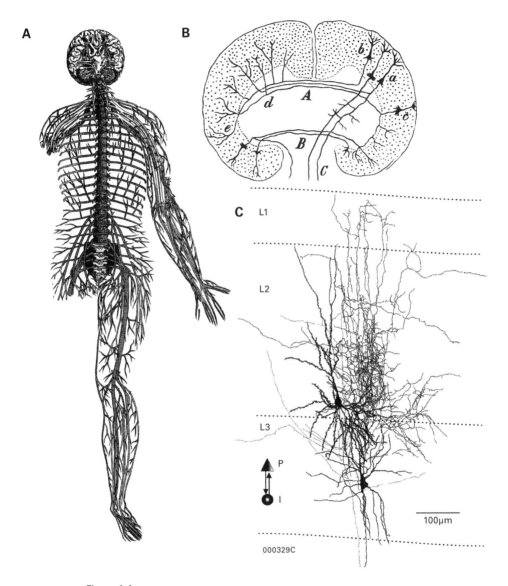

Figure 1.4
Examples of brain networks. (A) An illustration of the human central and peripheral
nervous system, from Andreas Vesalius's 1555 edition of *De humani corporis fabrica*,
reproduced from Swanson (2007) with permission. (B) A schematic diagram of the major
connections of the cerebral cortex, including commissural fibers linking the cerebral hemispheres, association fibers linking cortical regions, and fibers linking cortical and subcortical
regions. A, corpus callosum; B, anterior commissure; C, pyramical tract; a, b, c, cortical
neurons; d, e, axonal branches. Reproduced from Exner (1894). (C) Dendritic and axonal
arbors of a synaptically connected pair of neurons in cat cortex. At the bottom (dark gray)
is an interneuron (I) located in L (layer) 3 whose axon innervates a L2 pyramidal cell (P).
Scale bar: 100 μm. Reproduced with permission from Thomson et al. (2002).

nervous system, nodes most often refer to neurons or brain regions, while the edges between them can stand for a variety of measures of association, including the strength of a structural linkage (synapse, pathway) or an estimate of the dynamic flow of information. The variety of ways in which brain networks can be defined and measured is a somewhat unique feature compared to other fields—most applications of graph theory in social or natural systems so far have focused on fairly static representations without attempting to track dynamic network interactions. Dynamics, however, are an integral aspect of neural function, and thus dynamic networks represent a major branch of brain graph analyses. Broadly, brain networks can be classified as describing structural connectivity (anatomy), functional connectivity (statistical dependencies), and effective connectivity (causal relations) among collections of nodes (Jirsa and McIntosh, 2007; figure 1.5; table 1.1). Structural connectivity is the central objective of connectome-mapping studies while functional and effective connectivity describe the many facets of variable brain dynamics that accompany different aspects of sensorimotor function, behavior, and cognition.

Before observations of brain structure or function can be analyzed with the tools and metrics of graph theory, the empirical data must be represented in the form of a network (Bullmore and Sporns, 2009). Key steps in this process involve the definitions of nodes and edges. If the data come from neurophysiological recordings, network nodes might correspond to individual neurons, while neuroimaging studies require that the brain be divided into regions or parcels. This parcellation step is critical because many graph measures are sensitive to the way nodes (and thus edges) are initially defined. Parcellation strategies for the human brain are thus a central concern of current efforts to map the human connectome (see chapter 5). Once nodes are defined, their mutual pairwise association can be determined from measurements of structural, functional, or effective connectivity. These pairwise associations can be assembled in the form of a connection matrix, which, in turn, represents a graph or network. The edges between the nodes define the graph's adjacency structure, that is, they determine which nodes are immediate neighbors. Depending on the nature of the measure used to define the edges, graphs can be binary (edges are either present or absent), weighted (edges can take on graded values), undirected (edges express a symmetrical relationship), or directed (edges express an asymmetrical relationship). The graph adjacency makes no reference to the spatial position of the nodes and edges, instead capturing only the topology of the network.

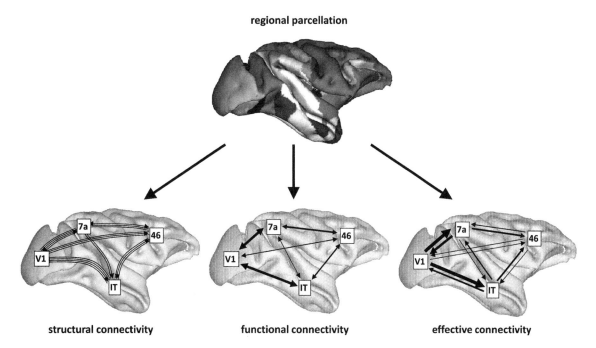

Figure 1.5
Structural, functional, and effective connectivity. This schematic illustration shows a lateral
view of the macaque cortex and illustrates the different modes of brain connectivity
through the relations between four cortical regions, V1 (visual area V1), 7a (parietal visual
area 7a), 46 (prefrontal area 46), and IT (inferior temporal cortex). The diagram at the top
shows a regional parcellation of the cortical surface, defining cortical areas and thus the
nodes of the brain network. Structural connectivity (left) is shown as a collection of white
matter fiber bundles, functional connectivity (middle) is shown as symmetrical statistical
relationships (arrows), which can be extracted from regional time courses of activation,
and effective connectivity (right) is shown as inferences of directed (causal) interregional
interactions. See figure 2.3 for a related illustration of the dynamic aspect of functional
connectivity.

As I will discuss later (in chapter 7), the spatial embedding of brain
networks entails a close relationship between the location of network
elements and their propensity for being topologically connected.

Graph theory offers a comprehensive set of quantitative measures that
capture global (network-wide) or local (node or edge specific) aspects
of connectivity (figure 1.6). Table 1.2 provides a glossary for a selection
of some of the most important graph concepts and measures that will be
referred to throughout the book. More in-depth and formal surveys of
graph measures are available in the form of numerous review articles
(e.g., Rubinov and Sporns, 2010; Kaiser, 2011). Applications of graph

Table 1.1
Major modalities of brain networks

Network Modality	Edge Representation	Empirical Techniques	Network Characteristics
Structural connectivity	Presence/absence of physical link (synapses, pathways), biophysical efficacy (synaptic weight), time delay (chapters 2, 3)	Microscopy: tissue volume reconstruction (chapter 4) Neuroanatomy: tract tracing (chapter 5) Neuroimaging: diffusion imaging/tractography (chapter 5)	Weighted or unweighted, sparse and directed (synapses, projections), sparse and undirected (diffusion MRI)
Functional connectivity	Statistical relationships between neural time courses (e.g., spikes, EEG, BOLD; chapter 6)	Neurophysiology: spike or field potential correlations EEG/MEG: correlation, synchronization, coherence, phase locking fMRI: BOLD signal cross-correlations, partial correlations (chapter 6)	Full and weighted, or sparse and weighted (or unweighted) after thresholding; undirected
Effective connectivity	Causality inference based on temporal precedence cues; causality inference based on generative model (chapter 6)	Spikes, EEG/MEG, fMRI: time series analysis (e.g., Granger causality, transfer entropy) or model inference (e.g., dynamic causal modeling)	Full or sparse; weighted (or unweighted) and directed

Structural connectivity is also referred to as anatomical or synaptic connectivity. The distinction between functional and effective connectivity is based on whether network edges are expressing directed influences. An alternative and more stringent definition of effective connectivity refers only to the explicit inference of a causal or generative model (e.g., Friston, 2011). MRI, magnetic resonance imaging; EEG, electroencephalography; BOLD, blood oxygen level dependent signal; MEG, magnetoencephalography; fMRI, functional magnetic resonance imaging.

theory to the brain are covered in some detail in Sporns et al. (2004), Bassett and Bullmore (2006), Stam and Reijneveld (2007), Bullmore and Sporns (2009), Guye et al. (2010), Wang et al. (2010), Bullmore and Bassett (2011), Telesford et al. (2011), Sporns (2011a), and Stam and van Straaten (2012). An open-source Matlab toolbox for computing all of the measures discussed in this book, including a number of brain connectivity data sets, is available at www.brain-connectivity-toolbox.net.

The most fundamental graph measure is the node degree. It refers to the number of connections that are attached to a specific node. Many other graph measures are derived from or correlated with node degree, and some of the local and global architectural features of a network can be gleaned from its degree distribution. A related measure is the "weighted degree," or node strength, which in a weighted network

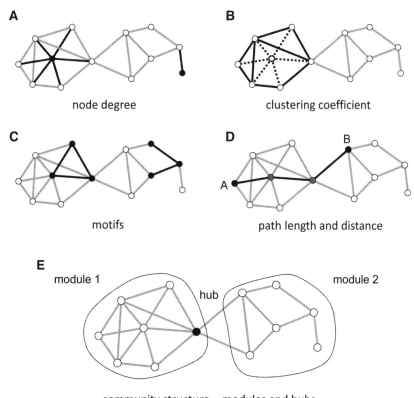

Figure 1.6
Network measures. This schematic diagram shows a selection of some measures that are among the most widely used in neuroscience. The measures are illustrated in a rendering of a simple undirected graph with 12 nodes and 23 edges. (A) The node degree corresponds to the number of edges attached to a given node, shown here for a highly connected node (left) and a peripheral node (right). (B) The clustering coefficient is shown here for a central node and its six connected neighbors. These neighbors maintain 8 out of 15 possible edges, yielding a clustering coefficient of 0.53. (C) The network can be decomposed into connected subgraphs, also called network motifs. The plot shows two examples of two different motifs composed of three nodes. (D) The distance between two nodes is the length of the shortest path. Nodes A and B connect in three steps, through two intermediate nodes (shown in gray). The average of the finite distances for all node pairs is also called the graph's path length. (E) The network forms two modules interconnected by a single hub node. Reproduced with permission from Sporns (2011b).

Table 1.2
Important graph concepts and measures that are widely used in the analysis of brain networks and are frequently referred to in this book

Graph Concept	Definition
Graph	A graph is a set of nodes and edges describing or representing a network.
Network	A network is a system composed of interconnected elements that can be mathematically represented as a graph. The terms "network" and "graph" are often used interchangeably.
Node	An element of a graph or network. In the case of a brain network, nodes may represent a neuron, a neuronal population, a brain region, a brain voxel, or a recording electrode. Nodes are sometimes also referred to as "vertices."
Edge	Nodes are linked by edges (also called links or connections). Edges may be directed or undirected, and they may be binary or have fractional weights.
Topology	The geometric relation between nodes defined by their connecting edges, irrespective of any metric distances or spatial embedding.
Binary graph	A binary graph contains only binary edges, that is, it records only whether a pair of nodes is connected or not. If a connection is present, the edge is set to 1; otherwise it is 0. Binary graphs can be directed or undirected. Binary graphs often result when a threshold is applied to continuous data matrices.
Weighted graph	A weighted graph contains edges that can take on any fractional value (including positive and negative values).
Undirected graph	All edges in an undirected graph represent a symmetrical relation between each pair of nodes—for example, a cross-correlation.
Directed graph	Edges represent asymmetrical (directed) relations between node pairs—for example, a synaptic link or a causal effect.
Path	A path is a set of unique edges that link one node to another. In directed graphs, paths consist of sets of directed edges that link a source node to a target node. In most graphs, a large number of paths exist between any pair of nodes.
Distance	The distance refers to the length of the shortest path between a given pair of nodes. If no path exists, the distance is infinite. Distance is recorded as the number of distinct edges (an integer) in binary graphs or as the combined lengths of the edges comprising the path in weighted networks. Distance refers only to the topology of the graph, not its metric or spatial embedding.
Connection matrix	The most basic representation of a graph or network in matrix format, with the entries a_{ij} of the matrix equal to the weight of the connection between node i and node j. The entries a_{ij} are zeros or ones for binary graphs. In binary graphs, the connection matrix is also referred to as the adjacency matrix.
Distance matrix	The entries of the distance matrix contain the distances between all pairs of nodes.
Module	A community of nodes, generally defined by the connection topology. Modules tend to comprise nodes that are more strongly interconnected within than between modules. In brain networks, modules may be defined on the basis of structural or functional connections.
Hub	A node that has high influence or importance to the integrity of the network and its global interconnectedness. Hubs can be detected on the basis of their high degree or high centrality.
Core	A network core is a coherent set of nodes that are highly and mutually interconnected. A core can be mapped by using a recursive procedure that prunes away weakly connected nodes (i.e., nodes with low degree).

Table 1.2
(continued)

Graph Concept	Definition
Rich club	Related to the core, a rich club is a set of high-degree nodes that are more strongly interconnected than expected by chance.
Random network	A network whose nodes are randomly interconnected. In the simplest case, a random network is generated by assigning edges to each node pair with a fixed and uniform probability. More complex random models can be constructed.
Small-world network	A network whose average clustering coefficient is similar to that of a regular lattice network and whose characteristic path length is similar to that of a random network.

Graph Measure	Definition
Degree	The most fundamental attribute of each node, referring to the number of edges (undirected or directed, i.e., incoming and outgoing) that are attached. Across the whole network, statistics on node degrees are often summarized in a degree distribution.
Strength	The sum of all edge weights (incoming and outgoing) for all edges attached to a given node.
Clustering coefficient	The fraction of edges (out of all possible) that connect the neighbors of a given node. The clustering coefficient of a node captures the degree to which its neighbors are also neighbors of each other (the "cliquishness" of a network neighborhood). The clustering coefficient can be averaged across an entire network. Different versions of the measure exist for undirected and directed, binary and weighted graphs.
Path length	Computed from the distance matrix, the path length (also called "characteristic path length") is the average of all finite distances in a network.
Modularity	The modularity score is computed relative to a partition of the network into modules. For a given partition, the modularity score records how many of the graph's edges are made within the modules, relative to what would be expected by chance. The modularity of a graph represents the optimal score that can be achieved under any partitioning scheme.
Global efficiency	The global efficiency is the average of the inverse distances across a graph. If two nodes are unconnected, their inverse distance is 0. In binary networks, the efficiency of an unconnected graph (no edges) is 0 and the efficiency of a fully connected graph is 1.
Centrality	In general, centrality expresses the importance or influence of a given node or edge. There are many measures of centrality. For example, the node betweenness centrality is computed as the function of short paths between all nodes of the network that pass through a given node. An equivalent measure can be computed for all edges.

These definitions are deliberately simplified and nonmathematical as they are meant to provide an intuitive idea and a first point of reference for the nonspecialist reader. For more in-depth treatment and mathematical background (including primary citations for all measures), see Rubinov and Sporns (2010).

records the sum of the weights of all connections maintained by a given node. The importance of node degree and strength derives from the fairly direct impact of degree on the dynamic "importance" of a given node. "Importance" captures the extent to which a network element has access to the rest of the network, influencing or affecting inter-actions elsewhere. Other measures of influence, such as various cen-trality measures (e.g., closeness centrality, betweenness centrality, eigenvector centrality) are often found to be correlated with node degree or strength.

Graph measures relevant to the brain can be divided into three catego-ries by virtue of what they tell us about brain organization. Measures of segregation capture the degree to which the nodes of a network exhibit clustered connectivity, which arises, for example, when connected part-ners (neighbors) are also neighbors of each other. The clustering coef-ficient of the network, generally expressed as the mean of the clustering coefficient over all nodes, is high if many of its connected nodes have common partners. Of particular interest are networks that can be decom-posed into distinct communities or modules, defined on the basis of the density of connections within and between modules. Measures of integra-tion estimate how efficiently information can be exchanged among all nodes in the network. Commonly used metrics to express this capacity are the path length and the global efficiency. Measures of influence yield metrics for individual nodes and edges—for example, quantifying their contribution or participation in dynamic processes unfolding on the network. Examples are measures of centrality, which is an important indicator of hubs in the brain. Most network measures, once obtained from empirical data, must be compared to appropriate random models— for example, randomly rewired networks that have equal size, edge density, and node degrees—to assess their significance. In general, the full characterization of a given network in terms of its topology, the dif-ferent network roles of nodes and edges, and its overall architecture requires the evaluation of a broad range of network measures. As it turns out, many empirical networks, including those found in the brain, express characteristic combinations of network attributes that are associated with specific topological families.

The modern era of network science began with the realization that virtually all real-world networks exhibit highly nonrandom properties of local and global patterns of network connectivity. A number of these properties were found to be universal in the sense that they could be identified across a wide range of natural, social, and technological systems. Among these, the "small-world" property is of particular interest to neuroscience. The small-world phenomenon, long studied in the context of social networks (Travers and Milgram, 1969), refers to the surprising tendency of some very large networks to allow links between any two nodes via short paths, or sequences of a small number of unique edges. A large social network with thousands or millions of nodes (people) often contains a remarkable number of very short paths of acquaintance-ship that link most people to each other.[10] Duncan Watts and Steven Strogatz, in a seminal paper published in 1998, noticed the joint occurrence of two topological attributes, short paths and high clustering, across a wide range of networks, from collaborations among movie actors, to the U.S. power grid, to the synaptic connectivity of the nematode *Caenorhabditis elegans* (Watts and Strogatz, 1998). Soon after, small-world architectures were also found in structural connectivity data recording large-scale projections among regions of mammalian cerebral cortex (Sporns et al., 2000; Hilgetag et al., 2000; Sporns and Zwi, 2004).

Closer examination reveals that small-world attributes like high clustering and short path length, despite their near-universal presence, do not identify a single coherent topological class. Rather, it is possible for networks to attain small-world connectivity in different ways. Structural and functional brain networks express small-world attributes through the existence of modules or communities of tightly interconnected nodes that are more weakly coupled among each other. In many cases, these modules are arranged hierarchically (as "modules within modules"), an architecture that may have important consequences for neural dynamics (see chapter 7). The detection of network modules or communities is of special importance for studies of brain networks as it allows the identification of closely coupled subnetworks and functional systems. We will encounter modules repeatedly throughout the book in various contexts, including when discussing the parcellation of the brain into coherent regions (chapter 5), the identification of functional networks supporting different cognitive capacities (chapter 6), and the definition of global network architecture (chapter 7).[11]

While most network approaches can, in principle, be applied to network data regardless of origin, careful distinctions have to be made in the interpretation of network metrics obtained from structural and functional brain networks (see chapter 6). Structural networks are considerably more straightforward to define and interpret because of the sparsity and specificity of their links and their (relative) stability across time. Functional networks exhibit significantly greater temporal variability and comprise statistical relations between neurons or brain regions that may or may not be structurally linked. These specific characteristics of structural and functional networks entail differences in the way these networks are analyzed.

In summary, network theory offers an indispensable framework for the representation and analysis of connectome data sets. Extending a gradual shift in emphasis from functional localization to functional integration (Friston, 2009; figure 1.7), the growth of connectomics in systems neuroscience will be accompanied by an expansion of graph-based modeling and data analysis. Importantly, network theory offers an extremely broad theoretical framework that transcends the traditional boundaries of scientific disciplines and links neuroscience with the emerging science of complex systems.

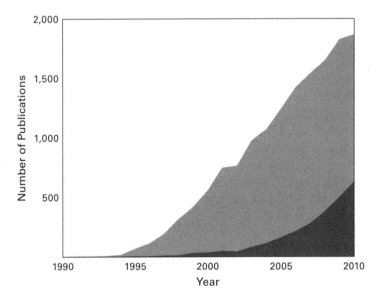

Figure 1.7
The shift from brain activation to brain connectivity. The graph shows an estimate of the number of neuroimaging publications per year that focus on activation (functional segregation, light gray) and connectivity (functional integration, dark gray), respectively. These estimates were derived from a search of the ISI Web of Knowledge with the search terms "((neuroimaging OR fMRI OR DTI) AND activation)" and "((neuroimaging OR fMRI OR DTI) AND connectivity)." The proportion of papers referring to aspects of functional integration has risen from less than 5 percent in 2000 to around 30 percent in 2011; their number has grown over 20-fold. Based on a similar figure first published in Friston (2009).

An "ome" for Neuroscience

The discovery of the human connectome will bring significant new opportunities to brain sciences. The connectome is a foundational neurobiological data set, a structural model of the brain that is indispensable for understanding brain function. Like other structural models in biology, the connectome provides a basic plan, a necessary ingredient for building mechanistic models of brain activity. However, while necessary, the connectome alone is not sufficient for understanding neural dynamics and behavior. The relation of structure to function, centrally important all across biology, is complex and nonlinear. The connectome is a key player in constraining and shaping neural activity, but, as we will see in later chapters, knowledge of the graphical layout of the connectome is only a first step toward a comprehensive account of brain function. Deep understanding of the connectome can only come from considering brain networks in the context of the whole organism and its behavior.

The connectome offers a common operational goal for a broad spectrum of neuroscientists working across different scales and systems. In the future, connectomics will likely foster increased collaboration and cooperation between researchers who previously worked in relative isolation from one another. Connectomics is an inherently transdisciplinary endeavor that brings together anatomists, neurophysiologists, radiologists, geneticists, and computer scientists. Like systems biology, connectomics employs a blend of hypothesis-driven and discovery-based research that involves the integration of multiple data types. Connectomics culminates in the construction of quantitative computational models that embody neurobiological mechanisms at multiple levels of organization. As connectomics gains ground in neuroscience, it supplements more conventional small-scale (single-laboratory) research with a model now commonly seen in the physical sciences: very large-scale projects that are driven by consortia of experts aiming for broad research objectives and clearly defined deliverables while building technologies and infrastructure that benefit entire research communities. This model naturally involves interdisciplinary collaborations, with greater dependence on specialized technical expertise and a complex management structure. In addition, it strongly relies on informatics resources with the explicit goal of cumulative data collection and data sharing (see chapter 8). Connectomics represents one of the first examples of this research model in neuroscience.

In 2012, several concerted research efforts directed at discovering the human connectome are under way. In the United States, the National Institutes of Health supports two large multi-institution research consortia through the Human Connectome Project (http://humanconnectome. org/consortia/). Awarded in September of 2010, one grant supports work led by Washington University and the University of Minnesota (in addition to seven other institutions) involving the study of structural and functional brain connectivity, as well as behavior and genetics, of 1,200 participants. Separately, a second grant supports the development of new imaging technology and analysis tools for structural brain connectivity, centered at the University of California (Los Angeles) and Massachusetts General Hospital. Other efforts, some of them in Europe and Asia, are rapidly gathering momentum.[12] In addition to human connectome projects, several large-scale efforts are under way to map the connectome of the mouse brain (e.g., http://www.mouseconnectome.org/; http://brainarchitecture.org/) and of the fruit fly *Drosophila* (e.g., http:// www.flycircuit.tw/; http://research.janelia.org/Chklovskii/). Not surprisingly, a key focus of many of these projects is technology development, leading to methodological enhancement and validation. The science itself will accelerate as new methodologies are shared across laboratories and become more affordable and reliable. The inexorable rise of computation in the biological sciences further fuels progress in the acquisition and analysis of connectome data sets. Despite the many challenges that accompany efforts to map the connectome of any species, comprehensive network maps of the brains of several "model organisms" will become available at an accelerating rate and with ever-increasing resolution and accuracy.

Connectomics is an exciting new field, but a sober assessment of its future promise is in order.[13] I share the enthusiasm of many early practitioners in this emerging field, but I am also keenly aware of the significant difficulty of relating a structural map of the brain to neural dynamics, computation, cognition, and behavior. The project of mapping the connectome is sometimes referred to as tracing the brain's blueprint or wiring diagram, and the resulting map is widely viewed as central for making us who we are as a species and as individuals. The simplicity of this idea is, at first, rather appealing.[14] However, serious problems arise when the notion of "wiring diagram" is taken too literally. The brain is not a giant electrical appliance, or a powerful computer chip, whose wiring is engineered to carry out specific operations. I believe a different perspective is needed to make sense of the intricate web of trillions of synaptic links that form a human brain. That perspective comes from viewing the brain as a network whose physical architecture enables *complex dynamic behavior* (Sporns, 2011a; Bassett and Gazzaniga, 2011). Brain networks operate as integrated systems where connectivity is laid out in the service of bringing about a wide range of global functional outcomes. The combined action of many individual elements and connections at small scales generates collective and coordinated states at large scales that are essential for cognition and behavior. In this dynamic sense, the network architecture of the connectome is critically important for enabling integrative processes in the nervous system.

Understanding integrative processes from the interactions of neural elements is a central research focus of connectomics, an extension of systems biology to the brain. A corollary of adopting this perspective is that brain function cannot be fully *reduced* to the connectome or wiring diagram, just as knowing an organism's genetic material does not furnish a complete account of its biological form and physiology. The connectome is not a blueprint of "who we are," no more so than the genome, which was supposed to deliver the "book of life" that explained "the chemical underpinnings of human existence" (Watson, 1990, p. 44).[15] Alas, despite the ever-increasing volume of genomic data, a principled understanding of how the genome underpins biological function is still in its infancy. Nevertheless, in ways that are subtle and complex, both genome and connectome carry important information about the natural history of the human species and the biological substrate of our individuality. Gaining access to the basic inventory of genetic components and a growing understanding of the complex networks they set in motion has transformed the biological sciences.[16] In a similar vein, discovering the human connectome will give us new insights and tools for asking better questions about how the structure of the brain gives rise to its functional operations, in both health and disease.

So far we have informally defined the connectome as a comprehensive description or map of the brain's connections. Now, let us explore the nature of the connectome in more detail—what do we mean by "connections," how are they mapped and described, and why does this description matter so much in neuroscience? What exactly is the human connectome?

2   What Is the Human Connectome?

The importance of synaptic patterns in neural circuits for brain function has been recognized for a very long time. The discovery of the specificity and diversity of the cellular architecture of the nervous system by Ramón y Cajal stands to this day as a towering achievement in the history of brain research.[1] Uncovering the anatomical connectivity of neuronal circuits and populations continues to be a central aim of cellular and systems neuroscience. Motivating modern research in this area is the hypothesis that mapping of anatomical circuits represents a fundamental step toward understanding brain function and physiology (figure 2.1). Cellular structure, and particularly connectivity, is widely seen as an important ingredient for enabling cellular computation, the specificity of physiological responses and their integration into coherent neural states. Until now, functional studies of cells and circuits have largely been carried out in the absence of detailed and specific information about the underlying connectivity. While the characteristic response properties of neurons such as orientation preference, selectivity for faces or objects, tuning to specific auditory frequencies, or reward prediction have been extensively studied, in virtually all cases a precise structural account of how these examples of functional specialization come about has remained elusive.

One of the major obstacles for tracing functional and physiological observations to the structural basis of the nervous system is the lack of a quantitative or comprehensive map of neural elements and their mutual connections. The creation of such a map is a principal goal of connectomics. Connectome mapping can be carried out directly, by deploying a broad spectrum of anatomical techniques (see chapters 4 and 5), or indirectly, by attempting to infer connections between circuit elements based on their temporal dynamics or functional responses. However, the inference of circuit connectivity from observations of

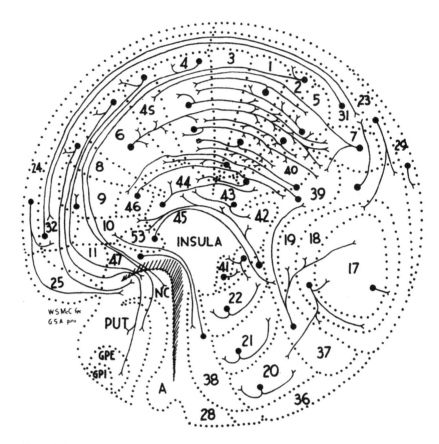

Figure 2.1
An early map of connections in cortex and basal ganglia of the Rhesus monkey (*Macaca mulatta*). The structures are arranged in a flat map with distinct cortical and subcortical regions presented in a manner that preserves their topological relations. Cell-like symbols indicate putative anatomical projections, identified by a neural stimulation technique called "neuronography." The creator of this map, the physiologist and theoretician Warren McCulloch, commented on its basic rationale: "Functional organization, which defines the temporal course of activity in any nervous mechanism, depends upon both physico-chemical reactions of constituents and their anatomical relations. Since reactions of all neurons are similar, it is frequently possible to deduce anatomy from observed activity or to predict activity from known anatomy." Numerals refer to Brodmann areas; NC, nucleus caudatus; PUT, putamen; GPE, globus pallidus, external segment; GPI, globus pallidus, internal segment. Reproduced from McCulloch (1944, p. 404).

neural time courses, from relations between physiological properties of neural elements, or from functional disruptions of circuitry following temporary or permanent lesions is indirect and subject to multiple types of error (see chapter 6). In contrast, directly mapped patterns of anatomical or structural connectivity between neurons are sometimes referred to as the "ground truth" necessary for mechanistic accounts of circuit dynamics and function.[2]

One of the central motivations for the connectome is to deliver the ground truth of circuit and systems anatomy. As it turns out, the origins of this goal go back at least several decades and have stimulated multiple parallel research efforts in different areas of neuroscience.

Multiple Origins, Common Motivations

In their seminal article describing the electron microscopy (EM) reconstruction of the nervous system of the nematode *Caenorhabditis elegans*, Sydney Brenner and colleagues formulated one of the key rationales for pursuing the complete connectivity pattern of an organism: "The functional properties of a nervous system are largely determined by the characteristics of its component neurons and the patterns of synaptic connections between them" (White et al., 1986, p. 2).[3] Implicit in this statement is a research program directed at the compilation of comprehensive brain-wide maps of neural connections, not only for *C. elegans* but for other species as well. The creation of the *C. elegans* map represented an early milestone of connectomics, an achievement that to this date has not been matched. *C. elegans* continues to be the only organism whose neural connectivity is completely known.[4]

Parallel and independent studies by neuroanatomists investigating the anatomical connections of nonhuman primate brains suggested a structural basis for the rich variety of observed physiological responses, particularly in the visual system. Semir Zeki's early studies of visual integration were based on the premise that "patterns of anatomical connections in the visual cortex form the structural basis for segregating features of the visual image into separate cortical areas and for communication between these areas at all levels to produce a coherent percept" (Zeki and Shipp, 1988, p. 311). Functional *segregation*, expressed in specialized physiological responses of cells and cortical regions, and functional *integration*, evident in coherent neural states underlying complex behavior, were both seen as dependent on the anatomical organization of cortical connections. Knowledge of the pattern of these connections would allow inferences about the structural basis of cortical responses and their integration.

A systematic effort to delineate the hierarchical arrangement of cortical areas as well as their organization into coherent parallel processing streams was carried out by Dan Felleman and David Van Essen, culminating in a landmark analysis of the connections of macaque visual cortex (Felleman and Van Essen, 1991). Summarizing the results of numerous anatomical studies reporting on interregional cortical pathways, Felleman and Van Essen were among the first to represent anatomical connectivity in the form of a connection matrix, a compact description of visual cortex that took the mathematical form of a directed graph.[5] Their analysis of macaque connectivity revealed several anatomical characteristics that had significant functional and physiological implications. Among them were the existence of segregated areas linked by distributed and mostly reciprocal connections, arranged into multiple overlapping processing streams, and a processing hierarchy extending over a number of more or less distinct hierarchical levels. Importantly, Felleman and Van Essen's analysis underscored the fundamental role of anatomical organization, that is, the system-wide arrangement of areas and connections (nodes and edges, in the language of graph theory) for an understanding of visual processing and computation. Further attempts at compiling comprehensive anatomical maps in other species followed, several of them with the explicit goal of creating neuroinformatics resources in the form of databases or repositories for the storage, annotation, and retrieval of connectivity data.[6]

The terms "connectome" and "connectomics" have multiple origins.[7] The first proposal to map the human connectome defined it as "a comprehensive structural description of the network of elements and connections forming the human brain" (Sporns et al., 2005). In parallel, Patric Hagmann, in his 2005 Ph.D. thesis, coined the term "connectomics" as the study of the brain's set of connections and noted that the brain's "computational power critically relies on this subtle and incredibly complex connectivity architecture" (Hagmann, 2005, p. 109; figure 2.2, plate 1). Other origins of the concept trace back to the work of researchers in cellular neuroscience and microscopy. Kevin Briggman and Winfried Denk argued for the necessity to extract neural connection matrices from detailed reconstructions of neural tissue recorded with EM because "knowledge of all the pre- and postsynaptic synaptic connections of a cell is necessary to understand its role in a network" (Briggman and Denk, 2006, p. 562). In the fall of 2007, Sebastian Seung, Jeff Lichtman,

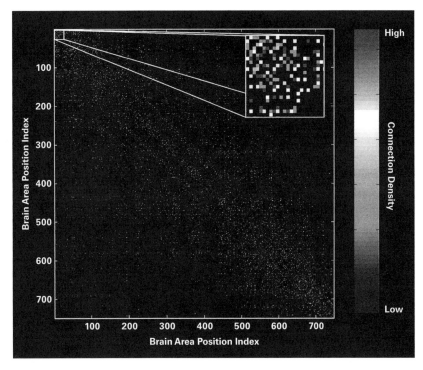

Figure 2.2 (plate 1)
The first picture of a human connectome. The image shows a graphical representation of human brain connectivity in the form of a connection matrix. Each of the over 700 rows and columns of the matrix represents a small patch of the brain's gray matter. The connection density between these patches is color coded. Note that much of the matrix is empty, reflecting the relative sparsity of large-scale interregional connections. Courtesy of Patric Hagmann (Hagmann, 2005, p. 110).

and Clay Reid organized a graduate seminar at MIT and Harvard entitled "Introduction to Connectomics," referring to connectomics as "an emerging field defined by the high-throughput generation of data about neural connectivity, and the subsequent mining of that data for knowledge about the brain."[8] In an article reporting on a novel neuronal labeling technique called *Brainbow*, Jeff Lichtman and colleagues defined "connectomic maps" as "connectivity maps in which multiple, or even all, neuronal connections are rendered" (Livet et al., 2007, p. 56).

The parallel origin of the connectome as a key target for neuroscientific investigation in cellular and systems neuroscience is remarkable. It not only underscores the timeliness of the idea but also affirms its potential transformative power in uniting scientific efforts that span vastly different levels of scale. All of the originators of the concept stressed the important role of structural connections, of connectional neuroanatomy, for shaping dynamic or functional responses of neural elements, ranging from those of individual nerve cells to entire brain regions. Also, there was general agreement that the essence of connectomics is the creation of connectivity maps of entire nervous systems that are as complete and detailed as technically possible. Thus, leaving aside for the moment some of the important differences that are intrinsic to various methodologies deployed at cellular or whole-brain scales (see chapters 4 and 5), a consensus definition of the connectome emerges: The connectome is a comprehensive map of neural connections whose purpose is to illuminate brain function.

It is worth underscoring this last point about the purpose of the connectome. The connectome is more than an accumulation of large amounts of empirical data. The real promise of the connectome derives from providing a mechanistic basis and a theoretical foundation for understanding the brain. An important additional step must be taken so that this promise can be fulfilled. Connectomics must include the development of analysis and modeling tools that reveal hidden regularities in the connection pattern and allow the formulation of predictive models of brain responses. An integral part of the original proposal for a connectome of the human brain was the idea that the connectome is a complex network that shapes brain function (Sporns et al., 2005; Sporns, 2011c, 2012). It is important to map and analyze this network because its connection topology contains rich information about architectural principles that underlie the expression of neural dynamics. The structure of the connectome also preserves a record of the organism's past. Connectivity is molded by the powerful forces of natural selection in evolution, and it is continually reshaped by development and experience. The connectome thus reflects the history both of the species and of the individual.

Embracing the connectome as a fundamental research goal implies a shift toward a connectivity- or network-based model of the brain. Network models are at the core of connectomics, and their adoption has far-reaching consequences for empirical and theoretical approaches to brain function. Before we explore structural and functional brain networks in more detail, the definition of the connectome requires some scrutiny. In the remainder of this chapter, we will examine some important conceptual aspects that articulate the idea that the connectome is primarily about *structure* (physical or anatomical connectivity) and that it is a *network description* of the brain.

Conceptual Foundations

The structural or anatomical connections of a nervous system form a finite set of physical links joining a finite set of neural elements. These physical links represent structural specializations of neurons that enable interneuronal communication, including most importantly all chemical synapses as well as electrical junctions. A number of structural parameters characterize these links. In the simplest case, a link might be characterized by a binary number indicating that the connection is present (1) or absent (0). More detailed representations of these links might record their number or density, their spatial attributes such as the physical location of the linked elements, the connection length and trajectory,[9] as well as cellular, biochemical, and biophysical properties that define the nature and magnitude of the link's physiological effects. All of these parameters are fundamentally structural in nature since they involve various aspects of neuronal and synaptic morphology, the cellular distribution of channels and receptors, and the biochemical modification of macromolecules involved in signal transduction and amplification. A complete and comprehensive structural description of a neural circuit or nervous system, a connectome, should include as many of these parameters as can be empirically determined. Recording which elements connect to each other, expressed as a set of binary relations forming an adjacency matrix, is only a first step. Additional structural information in the form of annotations that report on spatial layout and physiology should be linked to this binary map.

The emphasis on *structure* has several motivations. First, as discussed in the previous chapter, structure shapes biological function, and the fundamental importance of the connectome derives largely from an extension of this notion to neuroscience. Second, structure represents a definitive ground truth. The plausibility of connectomics rests on the fact that structural connections, a large but finite set of relations among neural elements, can be objectively verified and completely mapped. This aspect is unique to structural connectivity. In contrast, functional connectivity exhibits temporal fluctuations that strongly depend on context provided by internal state, sensory inputs, and cognitive demands (see chapter 6). These fluctuations give rise to an extensive set of functional networks that ceaselessly unfold across time, a set much larger than that formed by the underlying structural connections (figure 2.3). In addition, functional connectivity relies on a diverse range of methods for neuronal recording and time series analysis. Different methods for recording

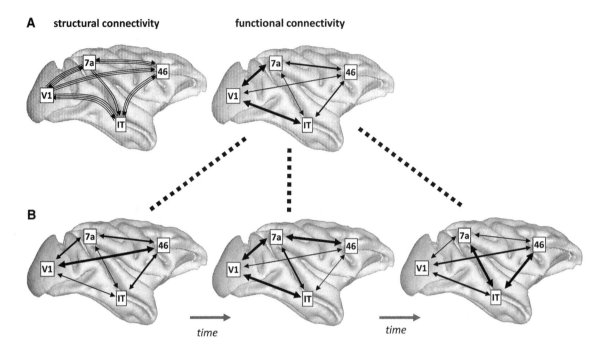

Figure 2.3
The dynamics of functional connectivity. The images represent a schematic diagram of the macaque brain (lateral view) and four brain regions: V1, visual area V1; 7a, parietal area 7a; IT, inferior temporal cortex; 46, prefrontal area 46. (A) Schematic illustration of structural connectivity and a longtime average of functional connectivity (cf. figure 1.5). (B) Functional connectivity changes across time. Each time point shows a changing network pattern of functional connectivity estimated from short episodes of neural recordings. The pattern in (A) represents an overlay or average of the many patterns seen in short episodes.

functional connectivity capture different aspects of neural dynamics, and there is no indication at the time of writing that a single universally agreed-upon method for measuring functional connectivity will soon emerge. Thus, fast-changing functional (and, by extension, effective) connectivity does not offer a clear point of convergence because it does not represent a finite and invariant set of elements and relations.[10]

Since structural connectivity is more stable across time (at least at the level of neural systems; see chapter 3) and because it is physical and veridical (in the sense that a physical link either demonstrably exists or it doesn't), different methods for measuring structural connections should converge on a common, or at least mutually compatible, connectivity layout. This point is important as it underpins one of the central claims of connectomics, its ability to furnish an objectively verifiable and invariant structural foundation for brain function. In principle, all methods employed for mapping structural connections should uncover an identical map. (In reality, this may be difficult to achieve due to methodological limitations such as resolution limits; see chapters 4 and 5.) Any disagreements between different methods should be resolvable by further refinement and continued observation. Once a comprehensive structural map has been drawn, the first principal aim of connectomics has been achieved.

And yet, however detailed this map may be, it would represent only a first step toward understanding how structural connections give rise to brain dynamics and behavior. An analogy with genomics may help to clarify this important point about the necessity, and at the same time insufficiency, of structure. Whole-genome mapping involves the sequencing of very large molecular structures, the polynucleotide strands of DNA. This structure provides full information about the catalog and arrangement of functional genomic units, an inventory of genes coding for proteins in addition to important noncoding regions and regulatory sequences. The mapping of these functional units was the principal aim of the Human Genome Project. However, the structural map that resulted from this large-scale research effort does not translate in simple ways to a complete understanding of "functional genomics." For example, the level at which specific genes are translated and expressed strongly depends on genetic, cellular and environmental context. Gene regulation relies on complex spatiotemporal networks that are still only incompletely understood. Hence, genetic sequences are only a first step toward delivering an account of the workings of functional systems. Quite analogously, the first goal of connectomics is to uncover a finite set of structural elements and connections that inform us about how to decompose the brain into functional units. Taking the next step and attempting to "decode" this structural map, or determining its role in the operation of the brain at the level of cells and systems, requires the consideration of a multitude of complex dynamic and functional interactions. Hence, knowledge of the connectome is necessary but not sufficient for understanding the brain.

This comparison with genomics leads us to a second important aspect of the connectome—it is a *description* of connectivity designed to reveal brain architecture. The term "description" implies data compression and reduction such that information about the described structure is maximized. In other words, a description relies on a way to decompose the structure into meaningful elements and their relations. Again, genomics offers an instructive comparison. Genomic sequencing was significantly aided by knowledge of the genetic code, which specifies how DNA structure is translated into functioning macromolecules. The genetic code helped to parse genomic sequences into meaningful architectural elements. Connectome mapping would greatly benefit from a set of principles that define how neural elements and their connections translate into building blocks of brain architecture, a compact description of brain connectivity. The connectome, defined here as a description of brain architecture, goes far beyond the collection of "raw data" by offering important information about connectivity in the form of structural patterns and regularities. A description is more than a list of parts. To turn to an analogy, a useful description of the great pyramid at Giza will likely make reference to the main geometrical and architectural features of its design rather than offer a list of the dimensions and positions of the 2 million blocks of limestone from which it is built. Similarly, the human connectome is a description of brain architecture that goes beyond enumerating all cells, synapses, or brain regions, but also reveals their basic plan. The arrival of the human genome provided such a basic plan for the genetic material, thus grounding our efforts to understand the biological bases for human variation and our relation to other species. It also answered important questions about genomic organization, including the precise number of genes[11] and their structural arrangement and regulatory couplings. The basic plan of the human connectome will answer similar important questions about brain architecture—for example, the number of distinct and segregated cortical regions,[12] and their topological, spatial, and functional relations.

Are compact descriptions of brain architecture possible to achieve? At least at the larger scales of brain regions and systems, tangible progress has already been made (see chapter 5). At finer scales, the existence of meaningful compressed and statistical descriptions of cells and circuits is very much a matter of debate (see chapter 4). On one side, proponents of complete cellular reconstruction approaches to the connectome reject statistical descriptions since they fail to capture specific nonrandom attributes of cell morphology and synaptic connectivity (e.g., Briggman and Denk, 2006). Implicit in this position is a strong preference for "dense mapping" of the connectome, that is, the assembly of a connection diagram by imaging and reconstructing all neural elements and synapses within an individual organism's nervous system "all at once."[13] On the other side, alternative proposals are based on statistical features of "canonical" neural circuits that define the connection probabilities of relatively few types of excitatory and inhibitory neurons (Douglas et al., 1989; Douglas and Martin, 2004).[14] The idea of statistical descriptions of elementary circuits implies that EM reconstructions may be useful for determining and verifying connection probabilities or other statistical rules but that dense reconstructions of all cells may not be necessary for an understanding of the functioning of nervous systems at larger scales. The controversy will eventually be resolved through connectome-mapping studies that probe neural connectivity for statistical regularities.

Finally, I should reiterate the fundamental premise that the connectome is a description of a *network* (see chapter 1). As I discussed at great length, the essence of connectomics is the mapping of structurally defined neural elements and their mutual connections. Thus, connectome data sets naturally take on the mathematical form of networks and graphs. This places connectomics into the context of modern research on complex networks, including those intensively studied in other areas of biology. The relation to network science allows connectomics to capitalize on sophisticated theoretical and analytical techniques for characterizing the structure and operation of complex systems. In doing so, studies of the connectome will make a major contribution to laying a new theoretical foundation for integrative neuroscience. I will expand on the computational aspects of connectomics more fully in later chapters (chapters 7 and 8; see also Sporns, 2011a).

Once again, it might be helpful to draw a comparison between connectomics and genomics. At first glance, the network aspect of the connectome seems to set it apart from the linear text-like format of information encoded in the genome. In fact, superficially, a genome sequence is linear and one-dimensional, in humans forming a molecular string of roughly 3 billion base pairs. However, genomic information can also be viewed as creating networks of dynamic relations between elements where relations may be defined as coexpression or participation in similar functional contexts. Other types of relations result from the fact that genetic elements are placed and associate in physical space. Recent work on the spatial configuration of chromatin in the cell's nucleus suggests that physical interactions among DNA sequences reflect organized patterns of gene expression (Rajapakse and Groudine, 2011).[15] As we will see later in the book, this relationship between spatial organization and functional expression is common to both genome and connectome. Spatial proximity among elements defines functional domains for gene expression, and it is a strong predictor of connectivity and functional relations in neural systems as well (see chapter 7). Not only do genome and connectome represent or "store" abstract information but they are also physically embedded objects that operate in space and time, weaving complex patterns of self-organization.

Form Follows Function

Louis Sullivan's modernist dictum "form follows function" encapsulated functionalism in architecture by suggesting that intended functions precede their realizations in architectural forms.[16] The movement was built on a teleological view of function as embodying a "purpose" to which the physical form of objects (or organisms) is mere accessory. On the surface, this notion cannot be reconciled with the mechanistic view that pervades modern biology according to which biological structure comes first, as the substrate and origin of functional processes, be they actions of macromolecules or organismic behavior. And yet, given that functional outcomes are subject to selection pressure, which, in turn, has consequences for structural alterations, function can be said to constrain the envelope of possible structural designs. Recognizing the mutual dependence of form and function, Sullivan's protégé Frank Lloyd Wright developed an organic view of architecture whose guiding principle became "form and function should be one."

In the same vein, can the connectome serve as a building block for a more organic and integrative understanding of brain function? Its claim to promote such understanding rests on the dual premise that the connectome captures structural patterns that are objectively verifiable (approximating ground truth) and that it underpins the functioning of neural circuits and systems. The latter idea strongly motivates connectomics as an indispensable foundation for mechanistic hypotheses and computational models of the brain. The connectome serves as a major constraint on such models because "every theory of how any neural computation works will have to be consistent with the measured connectivity" (Briggman and Denk, 2006, p. 568). Indeed, the construction of mechanistically detailed and predictive models of complex brain functions requires the firm grounding provided by a description of the brain's neural connectivity.

Structural connectivity is also necessary for a mechanistic understanding of behavior, including that of humans. Studying behavior alone cannot reveal the mechanisms by which the behavior was generated. Assuming that a mechanistic and causal understanding of how neural processes give rise to behavior is indeed desired, the study of human behavior alone cannot lead to such understanding. Many have advocated that to achieve this goal it is necessary to gather data on "neural correlates" that accompany specific mental and behavioral states.[17] However, every behavior is accompanied by a huge variety of neural processes at all scales, not all of which contribute equally. Thus, the identification of neural correlates that cause a specific functional outcome depends on the explicit formulation of a generative model (instantiating a mechanistic hypothesis) that can account for both neural and behavioral observations and predict new ones. The pattern of connections between neural elements is an important and necessary ingredient for any generative model designed to uncover the network basis of the behavior under study.

However, any simple-minded concept of the connectome as a static wiring diagram that determines function immediately runs aground as several critical challenges come into play. Connectomics must come to grips with the inherent multiscale architecture of nervous systems, and with their considerable variability across individuals and across time. It is to these important challenges that we turn in the next chapter.

3 Challenges

Mapping the connectivity of any complex nervous system encounters many challenges, starting with the enormous number of neurons and their synaptic connections, as well as their diverse morphology and functional heterogeneity. As connectomics begins to address some of these challenges, new opportunities arise for gaining insights into fundamental aspects of brain organization. Here we discuss three significant challenges for any current and future attempts to map the human connectome, posed by the multiscale nature of brain connectivity, by the inherent individual variability of structural connectivity patterns, and by their ongoing structural remodeling and plasticity. These challenges are related as the following thought experiment illustrates.

Assume we are in possession of a complete connectivity map of the brains of two individuals, a description of their connectome at synaptic resolution. How would we compare the two maps against each other? How much alike would the two brains be, and how would we quantify this similarity? Assuming we know each neuron's spatial position, morphological class, and connectivity, could we superimpose the two networks and determine areas of overlap and disagreement? Or is there a common reference point, a canonical human connectome to which all observations of individuals can be referenced? These are important questions since one of the major goals of connectomics is not only to deliver species-specific patterns of connectivity but also to assess individual structural variability. The problem is compounded if we consider the effects of structural change over time. If we could acquire the connectome of a single individual at different time points separated by an hour, a week, a year—how much of the network structure would remain constant? What changes might occur over time in the arrangement of neural connections, and what impact might these changes have on the brain's elementary and integrative functions?

The task of comparing connectomes between individuals and across time can only be addressed if the multiscale nature of human brain connectivity is taken into account. At larger scales, prominent anatomical characteristics are held in common across individuals, allowing alignment and comparison of multiple brains. These characteristics include macroscale features such as the anatomy of brain regions and gray-matter nuclei. At smaller scales, any attempt to establish one-to-one correspondence of single neurons across individual humans would be utterly futile.[1] While major features of neuronal cytoarchitecture are shared across individuals, no two nervous systems are exactly alike at the level of dendritic and axonal branches, or spines and synapses. Thus, statistical approaches are needed to allow between-individual comparisons at the microscale, perhaps utilizing descriptive graph measures of circuit topologies. Any attempt at comparing connectomes will greatly benefit from defining connectivity across scales, from neurons to populations, up to regions and systems, thus identifying the building blocks of the brain's multiscale architecture.

The Challenge of Multiscale Architecture

Distinct functional units capable of performing some elementary dynamic or computational process can be identified at all hierarchical levels on the basis of both anatomical and physiological criteria. Such functional units range from dendritic compartments to single neurons, microcircuits, specialized brain regions and extended system-wide networks. Importantly, no single scale occupies a privileged position in this hierarchy[2]— from a systems perspective, processes at all scales contribute to global functional outcomes that become manifest in cognition and behavior. The cellular scale of individual neurons and their connections is often viewed as fundamental for brain function. However, meaningful functional units exist not only at the level of individual neurons but also at larger and smaller scales. At smaller scales, the integrative function of single neurons is the result of elementary computations carried out in subcellular compartments and networked together through cellular morphology. At larger scales, single neurons cooperate in neural collectives that share common structural and functional attributes, engage in coherent patterns of neural dynamics, and generate specialized mutual information with each other and with the environment. Small and large scales interact, as large-scale patterns emerge from and coordinate small-scale interactions.

Given the estimated number of neurons ($\sim 10^{11}$) and number of synaptic connections ($\sim 10^{15}$) in the human brain, a complete map of the connectome at the microscale would be extremely sparse—fewer than one in a million (less than one ten thousandth of a percent) of all possible synaptic connections actually exist. Visualized as a binary adjacency matrix, this map would contain a million zeros for every nonzero entry. Once such a map is created, navigating it would be greatly facilitated by identifying groupings or clusters of neurons that form anatomical or functional collectives such as local circuits, columns, nuclei, or brain regions. The application of clustering or dimension reduction methods to such a cellular connection matrix might reveal different scales of organization that appear as nested modules or communities of neurons. Clustering will gradually compress the description of the map by representing neural elements and their interconnections in a more economical manner—for example, as regions and interregional pathways at the large scale of brain systems. At these larger scales, the density of the connectome's network description increases. Neuroanatomical studies of the regions of the mammalian brain indicate that large-scale connection matrices contain around 20 to 40 percent (and perhaps as much as 60 percent) of all possible pathways.[3] Thus, connectome maps at different scales have radically different densities. These different scales form a nested hierarchy—smaller elements join together to form larger elements, which, in turn, form even larger elements, and so forth. As I will discuss in more detail later (in chapter 7; see also Sporns, 2011a), many of the integrative aspects of brain function depend on this multiscale structural arrangement of elements and connections. Thus, an important goal for connectome research is to accurately describe multiscale connectivity.

The lower end of this multiscale architecture extends all the way to subcellular structures. Individual neurons are not the smallest units capable of integrating complex signals or transforming inputs into outputs. Instead, evidence suggests that at least some elementary computations are carried out entirely within dendritic compartments. Subcellular structures such as dendritic branches can perform compartmentalized local computations (Polsky et al., 2004; London and Häusser, 2005; Branco and Häusser, 2010; figure 3.1). In a recent study, Branco et al. (2011) demonstrated that single dendritic branches of cortical pyramidal neurons can exhibit sequence-specific responses to patterned synaptic inputs. Thus, cellular morphology, including the branching pattern of dendrites and the spatial arrangement of synapses, may be crucial for

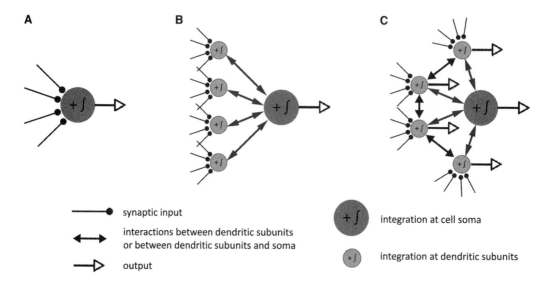

A **B** **C**

——● synaptic input

⟷ interactions between dendritic subunits
or between dendritic subunits and soma

⟹ output

+∫ integration at cell soma

+∫ integration at dendritic subunits

Figure 3.1
Dendrites as networks. The figure shows a schematic comparison of different ways to conceptualize neural processing in dendritic trees. (A) Traditional "point neuron" model, where synaptic inputs are integrated at the cell soma after applying a thresholded nonlinear function. (B) Two-layer network model (Poirazi et al., 2003), where synaptic inputs are locally integrated in dendritic subunits which are then integrated before a final output is computed. (C) Recurrent network model, where local release of neurotransmitters and neuromodulators allows dendritic subunits to generate their own output, and where dendritic subunits can mutually interact. Modified and reproduced with permission from Branco and Häusser (2010).

implementing elementary neural computations at a subcellular scale. By extension, higher-order computations such as those carried out by neurons can be thought of as resulting from the tree-like connectivity of dendritic compartments (Torben-Nielsen and Stiefel, 2009). Continuing work in cellular reconstructions may lead to the discovery of general graph-based combinatorial rules that govern dendritic computation in specific cell types.

Subcellular effects can play a decisive role in shaping the flow of information at the level of neuronal circuits. The placement of inputs on dendritic trees impacts the physiological efficacy of individual synapses, and spatial clustering of inputs on individual branches can result in synergistic effects on target neurons. The importance of dendritic microstructure and biophysics for controlling the effects of synaptic inputs on the integrative actions of a postsynaptic neuron has been extensively investigated in various cell types and in computational models. A convergent set of results suggests that synaptic inputs arriving from different neuronal circuits and systems occupy specific positions on the dendritic tree, which, in turn, determines the magnitude and the cooperativity of their effects on the postsynaptic neuron (e.g., Petreanu et al., 2009) and hence on the function of neuronal circuits. Mechanisms of neural plasticity, in part driven by network dynamics, can contribute to the emergence of subcellular compartments capable of carrying out specific nonlinear computation in individual neurons (Legenstein and Maass, 2011). These interactions of micro- and mesoscales are only incompletely captured in descriptions of connectivity that represent neurons as point-like entities.

Network elements are fairly straightforward to identify at the microscale of neurons and their cellular compartments. However, defining nodes and edges at larger scales requires the definition of anatomical or functional boundaries between large collectives of cells. The definition of coherent functional elements at the mesoscale of neuronal circuits and populations can be problematic, and there are numerous anatomical or physiological criteria whose application can result in different outcomes. Cell groupings in subcortical structures can often be identified by spatial proximity, coherent projections to other cell groups, or common neurochemical markers. In the cortex, a potential mesoscopic unit is the cortical column (Mountcastle, 1997). However, despite the widespread use of the concept in the cortical literature, there is little agreement as to the nature of the cortical column, except in highly specialized sensory regions such as the rodent barrel cortex. Columns are most frequently defined on the basis of physiological observations, but their structural boundaries are not clearly delineated (Rockland, 2010) and there are puzzling discrepancies between the spatial layout of functional properties and the known profiles of axonal and dendritic processes (da Costa and Martin, 2010).

A different concept points to elementary or "canonical" circuits as candidates for the basic building blocks of mesoscopic brain (cortical) architecture (Douglas et al., 1989). These circuits represent specific arrangements of excitatory and inhibitory neurons and their connectivity that can be characterized by connection probabilities between distinct types of cells arranged in separate cortical layers. This mesoscopic circuit element is thought to be reiterated throughout different cortical regions, with little structural modification, and thus represents a structural "building block" of the cortical architecture (Douglas and Martin, 2011). However, canonical circuits do not specify spatial modules, and they are not defined by discrete anatomical boundaries. Instead, their connectivity matrix describes a set of potential cellular interactions that can be dynamically reconfigured depending on inputs or past neural activity. Computation relies on circuit dynamics that is enabled by the anatomical pattern but does not reflect it in any simple way. The computational capacities of these transient functional circuits are still only incompletely understood, and the construction of detailed computational models and graph analyses are beginning to unlock the complexities of their dynamic operation (Binzegger et al., 2010). Canonical circuits, of different construction and composition, may also exist in other anatomical regions of the brain. It is important to note that the anatomical substrate for these circuits is fundamentally statistical rather than highly specifically wired. The empirical validation of statistical rules for the construction of elementary neural circuits will likely depend on results from dense connectome reconstruction efforts.

Structural segregation and functional specialization at the macroscale of regions and systems have been abundantly documented over decades of anatomical and physiological studies. Despite this abundance of evidence, the precise mapping of elementary units in terms of objectively defined structural boundaries still presents many challenges. To date, there is no universally agreed-upon chart or nomenclature of major anatomical subdivisions and interconnections for most of the human brain, including the cerebral cortex. Numerous criteria can be used for parcellating brain regions, including cytoarchitectonics, gene expression patterns, regional myelination, or patterns of anatomical and functional connections. Because of its importance for compiling large-scale maps of the human connectome, we will turn to the parcellation problem in much more detail later in the book (see chapter 5).

An important part of the parcellation problem is the need to characterize anatomical and functional brain regions in single individuals, due to the considerable individual variability of brain organization. This, then, is another significant challenge for connectomics, the variability of brain structure across individuals.

The Challenge of Individual Variability

No two human brains are exactly alike. This is certainly true if one attempted to align their individual neurons and synaptic connections. Statistical patterns may be preserved, but connectivity measured at the level of single neurons is highly variable across individuals both in terms of the number of elements and their connection topology. Even at the large scale, human brains exhibit significant individual variability for virtually all measurable features of brain structure. This extensive variability of brain structure across individuals is thought to be an important factor underlying measurable differences in brain physiology and dynamics, as well as in behavioral and cognitive performance.[4]

Structural variability is found at all spatial scales. At the cellular and synaptic level, there is significant structural heterogeneity among neurons and their interconnections both within and between individuals. Such variability is not limited to vertebrates; it is found even in "simple" and supposedly stereotypic brains of model organisms. In species like *C. elegans* whose cellular structure is derived from invariant lineage patterns in a sequence of stereotyped cell divisions, stochastic influences on embryonic and postembryonic development result in some degree of individual variation, including the spatial placement of cells and nuclei (Long et al., 2008) and their axonal wiring and synaptic contacts (White et al., 1983; Hall and Russell, 1991). Recent efforts to map cellular components and their interconnections in *Drosophila* have shed new light on patterns of individual variability in the fly brain. A detailed study of the fine-scale cellular morphology of local interneurons in the *Drosophila* antennal lobe revealed a surprising degree of individual variability (Chou et al., 2010). A systematic analysis of more than 1,500 cells allowed the identification of several morphological classes each characterized by coarsely stereotypic morphology. However, within each class, neurons differed significantly across individuals, both in their fine-scale structure as well as in their physiological properties. Commenting on this unexpected diversity, the authors concluded that "the wiring diagram differs considerably between individual fly brains" (Chou et al., 2010, p. 439), and they proposed that these variations may partly explain differences in behavior. With respect to the *Drosophila* connectome, these findings of structural variability "imply that the complete reconstruction of the wiring diagram of a single *Drosophila* brain will not yield a general wiring diagram for all *Drosophila* brains" (Chou et al., 2010, p. 448).

However, the observed heterogeneity of structural components across individuals does not necessarily result in widely divergent functional roles (figure 3.2). Overall, variable circuit elements contribute to neural circuits and systems in ways that are robust and result in functional stability. This functional homeostasis appears to dampen the impact of cellular heterogeneity and variability by allowing many different

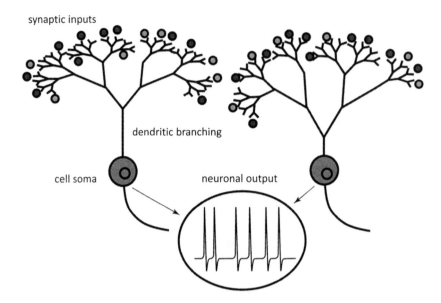

Figure 3.2
Neuronal homeostasis. Despite within- and between-individual variations in the number and arrangement of synaptic inputs and dendritic branching patterns, cells of the same morphological and functional type should produce a very similar dynamic output. Modified and reproduced with permission from Bucher (2009).

combinations of structural parameters to support nearly identical dynamic behavior (Tripodi et al., 2008; Goaillard et al., 2009; Marder, 2011). For example, detailed analysis of the leech heartbeat central pattern generator, a circuit comprising 16 neurons whose rhythmic output drives heart motor neurons, has demonstrated considerable functional consistency despite significant animal-to-animal variation in synaptic parameters (Norris et al., 2011). It appears that identical functional responses of neural circuits can result from disparate combinations of cellular parameters. Importantly, average parameter distributions may fail to fully characterize the richness of the underlying structural repertoire, thus motivating greater emphasis on capturing the true variability present within the population. The picture emerging from these studies is one where functional stability is not due to tightly controlled structural uniformity. Instead, structural variability in combination with as yet unknown compensatory mechanisms can yield globally consistent circuit dynamics. As Eve Marder has argued, these dynamics are more adequately described by families of models that differ in their structural parameters rather than a single model based on a composite of mean

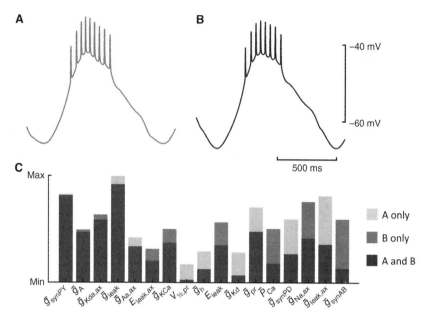

Figure 3.3
Similar dynamic behavior from different sets of neuronal parameters. The figure shows voltage-time traces (A, B) from two different instantiations of modeled lateral pyloric neurons of the lobster stomatogastric ganglion. Model parameters are shown in panel (C). Clearly, the two model neurons differ in multiple parameter settings but produce very similar voltage time courses. Other combinations of parameters are possible, and it is not obvious which combination of parameters (if any) is privileged. The model is described in Taylor et al. (2009); the figure is modified and reproduced with permission from Marder and Taylor (2011).

parameter values. Marder suggests that "we are entering an era in which we should attempt to collect as much data as possible on each individual, to attempt to see the correlations between underlying mechanisms and system behavior" (Marder and Taylor, 2011, p. 137; figure 3.3).

Variability is also found at the large scale of brain regions and systems. Significant differences in gross morphology of the human brain are immediately apparent, and they are readily found even when comparing brains of genetically identical individuals (figure 3.4). While many macroscopic features of brain anatomy (the relative positions and bilateral symmetry of key sensory and motor regions, the spatial layout of subcortical nuclei and the trajectories of major fiber tracts) are largely shared across individuals, other parameters such as the absolute and relative sizes of brain regions, the number and density of their constituent cells, and their axonal densities and biophysical properties all exhibit

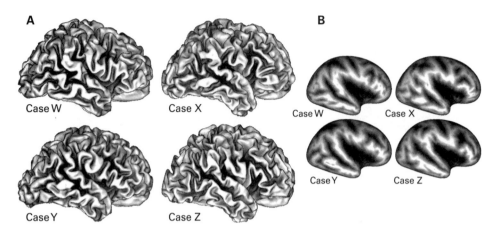

Figure 3.4
Individual variability in cortical folding. The images show right lateral views of four segmented cortical surfaces (A) and their corresponding sulcal depth maps (B), essentially
representing the depth profile of cortical sulci on a standard and inflated surface map.
Cases W and Y, as well as X and Z, are from genetically identical twins. Note the considerable variation of folding patterns across all four cases, including the twin pairs. Images are
from a study by Botteron et al. (2008) and reproduced courtesy of David Van Essen (Washington University School of Medicine, St. Louis).

significant variability. Individual human brains differ along many dimensions, including mass and volume, the folding pattern of the cortical
surface, the extent and spatial arrangement of cytoarchitectonic areas,
and the number and density of neuronal connections. For example,
numerous structural parameters across all stages of the human visual
pathway, from the retina to visual cortex, exhibit significant between-
subject variations. These include retinal cone densities (Curcio et al.,
1987), the size of pathways like the optic tract, and lateral geniculate
nucleus and V1 area and/or volume (Andrews et al., 1997).[5]

Many of these morphological features contribute to structural
variations in network connectivity. Combined analysis of anatomy and
behavioral performance suggests that these structural variations can partially account for individual differences in performance (figure 3.5).
Strong associations between structural brain measures related to gray
and white matter architecture and individual variations in behavior
extend from sensory perception and motor performance all the way to
complex cognition and aspects of consciousness (Kanai and Rees, 2011).
For example, in the human visual system, differences in cortical thickness
and gray matter density in specific regions of parietal cortex partially
predict differences in the temporal dynamics of bistable perception

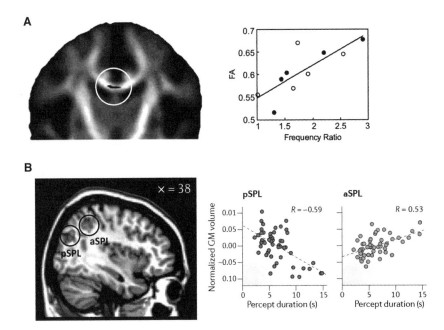

Figure 3.5
Correlations between brain structure and individual performance. (A) Relationship between white matter structure, measured here as the fractional anisotropy (FA), and the frequency ratio, a measure of performance in a bimanual finger-tapping task. Open and closed circles refer to females and males, respectively. Image modified (converted to grayscale) and reproduced with permission from Johansen-Berg et al. (2007). (B) Relationship between individual differences in perception and gray matter (GM) volume of two parietal cortical regions, the posterior superior parietal lobe (pSPL) and the anterior superior parietal lobe (aSPL). Longer duration of a percept in a visual rivalry task is positively correlated with a larger aSPL, but negatively correlated with a larger pSPL. Modified (converted to grayscale) and reproduced with permission from Kanai and Rees (2011).

(Kanai et al., 2010; see figure 3.5). These associations between structure and function can be explained by a combination of genetic and experiential factors. Heritability studies suggest that numerous structural brain measures, including aspects of white matter microstructure, are under genetic control (Glahn et al., 2007). Additional structural variability is the result of experience-dependent plasticity, which shapes the connectome at all scales from cells to systems (see below).

The high degree of structural variability at cellular scales poses a difficult problem for approaches to connectomics that target microscopic reconstructions of neural architecture. The reconstruction of a single connectome fails to capture patterns of individual variation and will not allow relating connectome data to differences in genetics and behavior. The problem is compounded by structural changes that accrue as a result of spontaneous and experience-dependent plasticity. Individual variation also calls into question strategies that rely on assembling connectomes through dense reconstruction of small tissue volumes sampled from multiple individuals since it will be impossible to combine them into a coherent high-resolution map. The challenge of individual variability can only be adequately met by the study of populations. Population studies of connectomes can capture variations in circuit topology and geometry present across multiple instantiations of nervous systems sampled from individuals of the same species. Population studies are also necessary for relating connectome architecture to genetics and behavior.

To be sure, structural variability also poses a significant challenge for large-scale neuroimaging approaches to the human connectome. However the impact of the problem is mitigated by the lower cost of acquiring these data from large populations and the greater phenotypic stability of connection topology at the large scale. Nevertheless, even at larger scales connectional variability is likely to be significant and the study of numerous individuals will be essential to relate variations of brain structure to function. This need to focus on individuals rather than on averaged or "standard" brains has many implications. Individual variability has, until now, not been a central concern of neuroscientific research. Instead, the focus has been on delivering descriptions of population averages, be they patterns of neural activations or behavior. Connectomics will usher in a major shift toward considering the structure of individual nervous systems, with a focus on how individual differences of network topology are predicted by genetic or environmental factors and, in turn, can predict functional variation. Connectomics carried out on populations of individuals thus provides a new source of rich information concerning the neural substrates of specific behaviors.

The Challenge of Remodeling and Plasticity

The cells and tissues making up an organism appear to have material permanence over long stretches of the organism's lifetime. And yet, virtually all of their constituent biomolecules are continuously replaced in a matter of hours, days, or weeks at the most. This rapid molecular turnover involves continual resynthesis of all structural elements of the connectome, including cellular and molecular components of neurons and synapses (Price et al., 2010).[6] Some of these components turn over with startling speed. For example, elements of the neuronal cytoskeleton such as actin filaments in dendritic spines have a half-life of around 40 seconds (Star et al., 2002). Important presynaptic proteins are removed from and reincorporated into synapses on a time scale of minutes (Tsuriel et al., 2006), and proteins comprising the postsynaptic density, a cellular structure important for plasticity, are replaced on a time scale of hours (Ehlers, 2003). As was recognized long ago, this rapid molecular turnover poses problems for the maintenance of molecular substrates of long-term memory (Crick, 1984; Lisman, 1985). The fluidity of the connectome at cellular and molecular scales requires control mechanisms to ensure stable dynamic outputs and functional homeostasis (see above).

At the somewhat larger scale of cells and synapses, significant changes continually shape and mold the connectivity of the nervous system by drawing on a host of mechanisms, from synaptic modifications to neuronal growth and structural plasticity. While most pronounced during early development, structural changes occur throughout the life span. An emerging view backed by increasing amounts of evidence suggests that the structural arrangement of neuronal circuits, including their connection topology, can undergo significant and rapid alterations even in the adult brain (Holtmaat and Svoboda, 2009). These alterations involve both dendritic and axonal compartments, and they have been observed in conjunction with learning and experience.

Earlier studies involving long-term observations of individual neurons and their dendritic morphology have suggested that larger dendritic branches of neurons in mouse barrel cortex remain stable over periods of weeks (Trachtenberg et al., 2002). However, while a significant proportion (about 50 percent) of dendritic spines were found to be stable over periods of a month, others were markedly transient and dynamic and exhibited both sprouting and retraction. Related observations revealed a gradual increase in the proportion of stable dendritic spines during development and into adulthood, as well as some regional differences in the extent of this form of experience-dependent plasticity (Holtmaat et al., 2005; figure 3.6). Specific changes in sensory inputs or behavioral training can alter the structural dynamics of spine formation and elimination. Hofer et al. (2009) examined the density and persistence of dendritic spines in mouse visual cortex in the course of monocular deprivation. Spine density in specific cortical layers receiving binocular sensory inputs increased following deprivation, and many dendritic spines formed during the deprivation episode remained stable even after the occluded eye was reopened. This suggests that structural modifications of dendritic

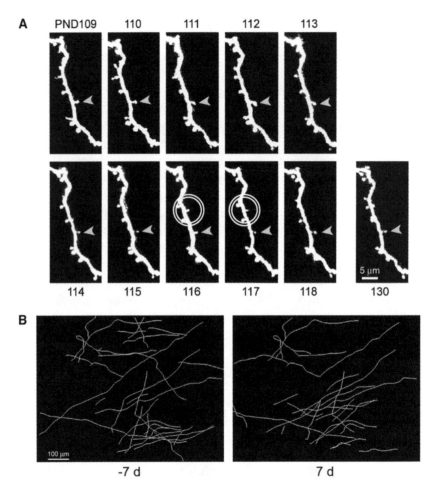

Figure 3.6
Structural remodeling of dendritic spines and axonal branches. (A) Time-lapse images of
a dendritic branch of a fluorescently labeled neuron located in adult mouse visual cortex.
Images are taken between postnatal day (PND) 108 and 130. The spine marked with a
white arrowhead remains stable over the entire observation period while the spine marked
by a circle appears and disappears. Modified and reproduced with permission from Holtmaat et al. (2005). (B) Tracings of axonal branches in adult macaque primary visual cortex,
7 days before (–7d) and 7 days following (7d) a focal binocular retinal lesion. The field of
view shown here is from the cortex surrounding the zone that receives inputs from the
lesioned part of the retina. Note that axonal segments change over time, with some segments appearing and others remaining stable or disappearing from view. Modified and
reproduced with permission from Yamahachi et al. (2009).

spines can outlast sensory experiences that triggered the change and may thus form a structural substrate for long-term retention of sensory memory. The formation of new spines following changes in somatosensory inputs or motor learning was also observed in mouse somatosensory or motor cortex (Yang et al., 2009). A percentage of newly formed spines remained stable over significant periods of time. A parallel and independent study by Xu et al. (2009) demonstrated the rapid generation of new spines in motor cortex following complex motor learning, with some spines forming within one hour of the initiation of motor training. Formation of new dendritic spines was associated with the practice of new, but not with previously acquired, motor tasks, supporting the idea that once-stabilized patterns of connections serve as a long-term basis for the retention of motor memories. In addition to spines, the branching patterns of dendritic arbors also exhibit some dynamic changes over periods of days and weeks, predominantly in GABA-ergic interneurons (Lee et al., 2005).

Structural dynamics of dendritic spines are mirrored by those involving the axonal compartment. A series of studies carried out in adult macaque primary visual cortex examined the structural stability and turnover of axonal branches and synaptic boutons in the absence of any overt changes in sensory experience or learning (Stettler et al., 2006), as well as under conditions where sensory inputs were perturbed (Yamahachi et al., 2009; figure 3.6). Using in vivo two-photon microscopy, both studies repeatedly imaged axonal branches and synapses of individual neurons over periods of several days and weeks. In the absence of external challenges, following axons and synapses over time revealed a surprisingly high rate of 7 percent per week for the turnover of synapses and concomitant changes in smaller-scale axonal branching patterns, while confirming the structural stability of larger-scale axonal branches (Stettler et al., 2006). The authors remark that "the turnover rate is surprisingly large, particularly if one considers the implications such a rate would have, if sustained and homogeneous over all boutons, for maintaining basic functional properties" (Stettler et al., 2006, p. 884). Whether this high rate of structural turnover is limited to a restricted subset of synapses or involves all of them uniformly is unknown.

Perturbations related to sensory experience can induce rapid bursts in the remodeling of cortical circuits. Numerous studies have documented specific physiological and structural changes in the course of perceptual learning (Gilbert et al., 2001) or in response to lesion damage in sensory pathways (Keck et al., 2008). Physiological observations show that neurons within a patch of cortex that has lost retinal inputs due to a binocular lesion regain responsiveness within hours and that their receptive fields shift to parts of the visual field represented in the surrounding unlesioned cortex (Das and Gilbert, 1995). Using in vivo fluorescence microscopy to track the morphology of individual neurons has now revealed substantial sprouting and pruning of axonal branches and synapses in adult macaque visual cortex following such lesions (Yamahachi et al., 2009). In concordance with physiological observations, cortical axons located in the area of the lesion exhibit significant sprouting and synaptic proliferation within just a few hours. Exuberant axonal outgrowth extends over several days and then gives way to axonal pruning, eventually returning to stable levels in the density of axonal branches and synaptic boutons. These rapid changes in cortical circuitry may be due to a temporary shift in the balance between addition and elimination of circuit elements observed during normal conditions. Additional evidence for rapid structural changes in connectivity following manipulations of sensory input comes from studies of thalamocortical synapses in the visual system of the mouse (Coleman et al., 2010). Here, analysis of EM micrographs demonstrate that significant synaptic remodeling of thalamocortical inputs immediately follows monocular closure, with synaptic densities decreasing by as much as 30 percent. Taken together, these studies indicate that alterations in structural connectivity—for example, synaptic rearrangements of sensory inputs following perturbations—can occur rapidly and are accompanied by changes in physiological responses. Structural alterations are not confined to periods of repair or recovery; they also occur at significant rates during normal functioning of cortical circuits.

In summary, while larger dendritic and axonal branches remain more stable, significant remodeling of smaller dendritic and axonal branches, including synaptic addition and elimination, occurs both spontaneously and in response to changes in input patterns. These structural changes take place on top of numerous biochemical and biophysical mechanisms for altering synaptic strength and efficacy. How can memory traces be conserved in light of the fact that the synaptic architecture appears to be very much in flux? One hypothesis states that long-lasting memory traces are preserved in stable structural arrangements of a subset of cells and synapses and that encoding of such traces involves mechanisms for memory allocation to specific neural elements (Silva et al., 2009). Another idea suggests that structural remodeling serves to alter connectivity between specific (and stable) circuits, thus modulating function (Chen and Nedivi, 2010). While there is evidence supporting the long-term stability of circuit elements such as dendritic spines following behavioral training (Yang et al., 2009), it is unclear whether ongoing circuit remodeling is truly limited to a subset of neurons or whether apparent structural stability and instability simply reflect changes occurring on different temporal scales. Even if individual spines or synapses can be shown to last throughout a large portion of an organism's lifetime, it is not clear how they can encode information about specific events or capacities if even a fraction of the surrounding connectivity exhibits significant structural alterations. In a system such as the brain, what individual circuit elements "stand for" is determined by the surrounding network. Despite the appeal of the idea that specific memories can be traced to individual spines or synapses, the integrative nature of brain networks and their remarkable propensity for structural change call this popular notion into question.

Further complicating the picture are possible fluctuations in connectivity due to global state changes of the organism. Recent studies on synaptic plasticity in relation to the sleep/wake cycle suggest the intriguing possibility that connectivity might exhibit rhythmic fluctuations. Patterns of gene expression, including genes involved in synaptic transmission, undergo significant changes in relation to the organism's behavioral state (Cirelli, 2009). Electrophysiological recordings from rat cortex indicate parallel changes in synaptic currents (Liu et al., 2010) and thus in synaptic plasticity. Size and volume of synapses can vary in relation to learning-induced changes in synaptic strength (Ostroff et al., 2010), raising the possibility of circadian variations in morphology of synaptic connections. A detailed study of cellular and circuit structure in *Drosophila* has shown that significant changes in spine number and the size of synapses occurs during waking and that these morphological parameters are renormalized during sleep (Bushey et al., 2011). The magnitude of morphological changes was found to be correlated with the richness of the wake experience. Whether these sleep/wake and plasticity-related effects have in impact on connection topology is currently unknown.

This dynamic picture of ongoing and experience- as well as state-dependent structural remodeling of neuronal circuits poses a major challenge for connectomics carried out at the microscale. Each dense connectome delivered by EM or light microscopy (LM) reconstructions (see chapter 4) represents only a snapshot of the microscale architecture of the nervous system, a still image of a dynamic pattern. Significant portions of the connection matrix delivered by microscale connectomics must be assumed to be highly variable, even within a single organism. This underscores the importance of identifying patterns that remain invariant over time and that can serve as the structural basis for stable functionalities of circuits and systems. These invariants are not likely to be found in individual structural elements, but in their spatial and topological arrangement and in global metrics of the network.

The developmental dynamics of the human connectome at the large scale are targets of intensive investigation, not least because a number of cognitive disorders are thought to have developmental origins. Several surveys of various stages of development in humans have begun to chart changes in network topology and organization, mostly on functional networks derived from fMRI (Fair et al., 2009; Supekar et al., 2009). These studies indicate that the functional architecture of the cerebral cortex is dominated by high clustering and modularity (i.e., higher functional segregation) at earlier developmental stages, while functional networks at later stages exhibit greater long-distance dynamic coupling and integration. Much less is known about the growth of structural connections in the human brain.[7] The application of diffusion MRI has begun to chart the genesis and maturation of brain connectivity from birth to early adulthood, in addition to a few reports on connectivity in utero (Kasparian et al., 2008). In a longitudinal study spanning the first two years of postnatal life, Fan et al. (2011) demonstrated that structural brain networks begin to exhibit small-world topology and nonrandom modularity even at very early developmental stages.

Studies that map structural connectivity with noninvasive diffusion imaging must take into account the changing composition of myelin and the resulting modulation of the diffusion signal. Myelin maturation plays an important role in rendering axonal pathways functionally effective by increasing their physiological efficacy and shortening conduction delays. The effect of increasing myelination on brain network topology was examined in a study of 30 individuals between 2 and 18 years of age (Hagmann et al., 2010b). The continuing maturation of white matter pathways was found to promote progressive increases in global efficiency and decreases in local clustering of brain networks while prominent structural hubs remained in place throughout this developmental period (figure 3.7). These structural changes are broadly consistent with a shift in balance from functional segregation to functional integration.

Structural change also accompanies the brain's response to physical trauma. Traumatic brain injury is often associated with damage to long-

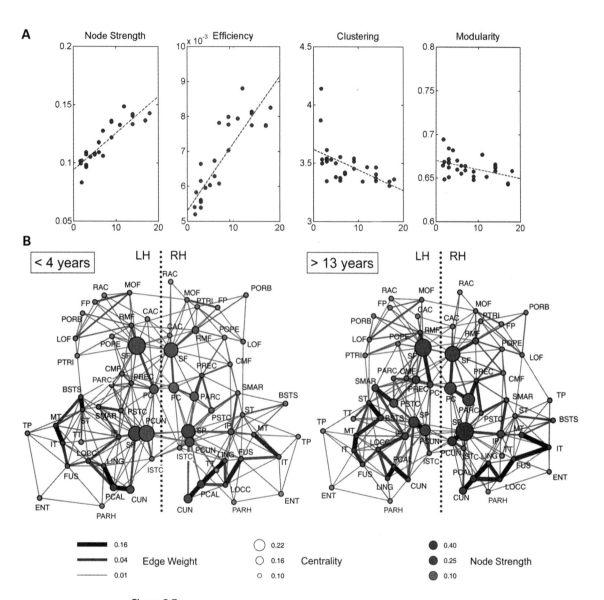

Figure 3.7
Development of cortical network topology. (A) Time course of average node strength, global efficiency, clustering coefficient, and modularity of human cerebral cortex, measured with diffusion imaging and tractography in 30 participants between the ages of 2 and 18 years. Significant increases in node strength and efficiency and decreases in clustering and modularity are due to the ongoing maturation of white matter projections in late development. (B) Hub regions, indicated here as highly central and strongly connected nodes, are in place during early development and continue to mature into adolescence. LH, left hemisphere; RH, right hemisphere; for abbreviations of brain regions please consult original publication. Data replotted from Hagmann et al. (2010b).

range interregional connections, and the extent of this damage is related to disruptions in behavior. A recent study by Kinnunen et al. (2011) provides evidence for a close association between cognitive impairment and the extent of axonal injury. The study also documents postinjury white matter changes throughout the brain, even in regions that are remote to the primary site of the injury. The distributed pattern of white matter abnormality was found to correlate with individual differences across patients in specific areas of memory and executive function. Structural changes in the brain's white matter not only result from brain injury but can also occur in the course of neurological recovery. Voss et al. (2006) reported ongoing structural modifications measured by diffusion MRI in a patient who underwent spontaneous recovery of some cognitive skills after many years spent in a minimally conscious state following severe head trauma. Changes in the diffusion signal were interpreted as due to axonal sprouting and regrowth, resulting in widespread changes in brain connectivity. These changes extended across several regions of cortex and correlated with behavioral improvements in several motor and cognitive domains. A more comprehensive longitudinal study of 30 adult patients who had suffered severe traumatic brain injury also documented progressive changes in the structure of cerebral white matter, the extent of which was correlated with outcome measures during recovery (Sidaros et al., 2008). The widespread effects of focal brain damage on the integrity of cortical networks was documented by Crofts et al. (2011) in a report on distributed changes in brain connectivity following stroke. Network analysis methods were successfully applied to identify brain regions and pathways with reduced centrality. Several of these regions were in parts of the brain far removed from the primary area of the stroke. Jointly, these clinical studies of brain injury and recovery reveal the complex relationship between the integrity of axonal pathways and cognition, and the potential role of specific changes in connectivity in behavioral impairment as well as functional recovery. Connectivity-based approaches (Grefkes and Fink, 2011) and connectome data will be essential for making progress toward mapping patterns of structural changes in patients as a tool for the development of novel diagnostic and therapeutic strategies.

Changes in white matter structure occur not only in response to brain injury but accompany changes in experience as well (figure 3.8). Scholz et al. (2009) first reported large-scale structural plasticity induced by behavioral training of a complex visuomotor task (juggling). Longitudinal measurements of fractional isotropy in white matter as well as gray

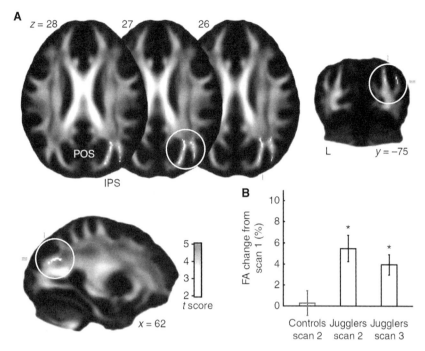

Figure 3.8
Large-scale structural changes following behavioral training. (A) Circled voxel clusters exhibit significant increases in fractional anisotropy between scan 1 and scan 2, acquired before and after a 6-week training period involving learning how to juggle. POS, parietal-occipital sulcus; IPS, intraparietal sulcus. (B) Summary data. Scan 3 was acquired after a subsequent 4-week period without juggling. FA, fractional anisotropy. Modified (converted to grayscale) and reproduced with permission from Scholz et al. (2009).

matter density exhibited localized changes in regions of medial occipital and parietal cortex. Such learning-related remodeling of the brain's white matter architecture may impact local and global network connectivity and thus offer a way by which individual experience can modify connectome topology. The possible relationship between individual experience and anatomical changes in brain connectivity suggests a structural basis for individual differences in behavioral performance (Johansen-Berg et al., 2010). Experience-dependent plasticity, in addition to genetic factors, may thus make a major contribution to the abundant structural variations present across individual connectomes, even at the large scale of brain regions and interregional pathways, and extending through development into adulthood.

Into the Jungle

The discovery of the human connectome faces numerous challenges. It is sometimes argued that these challenges, such as multiscale organization and individual variability (and others, not considered here in detail, such as the extraordinary degree of structural heterogeneity of neuronal types and synapses; Parker, 2010), render the connectome an impractical idea. The argument of impracticality is often raised when the connectome is considered in comparison to the genome, generally viewed as a much more tractable structure due to its linear arrangement in the form of a DNA sequence. However, a closer look at this comparison leads to the realization that some of the challenges facing connectomics have close parallels in genomics. First, despite the availability of genomes in the form of linear sequences,[8] the seemingly simple objective of identifying coding and regulatory sequences still presents a significant problem. Second, going beyond linear sequence information, genomes have a host of complex architectural features such as hierarchical (van Driel et al., 2003) and spatial organization (Parada et al., 2004) and the capacity for self-organization and pattern formation (Lieberman-Aiden et al., 2009). Third, genomes (within limits) can accumulate changes across an organism's lifetime as they undergo epigenetic modifications that reflect a history of environmental interactions (Richards, 2006). Fourth, genomic variability across individual organisms gives rise to variable phenotypes in ways that are still only poorly understood. Finally, the expression of gene products generates complex networks of protein–protein and metabolic interactions that unfold on multiple temporal and spatial scales. These complex networks are targets of ongoing research efforts in emerging fields like metabolomics and systems biology (chapter 1). Thus, while the first-order representations of genomes and connectomes share appealing simplicity (a string of letters, a matrix of ones and zeros), understanding their architecture and functional expression is demanding, to say the very least.

In addressing these challenges, network tools and network thinking are of particular importance. For example, network approaches are well suited for characterizing patterns of variability across individuals and for generating predictions about those aspects of individual variability that are most informative and most likely to result in significant differences in function and behavior. When observing networks across time—for example, during development—patterns of change can be reconceptualized as resulting from network dynamics, the interplay between developmental processes that shape human cognition and concurrent changes in brain connectivity that modify network topology. Similarly, variations in individual behavior can be related to variations in network architecture that are due to genetic factors or environmental influences. And detailed knowledge of structural connectivity allows the formulation of predictive and generative models for complex neural activity. The description of the human brain as a complex network can materially advance our understanding of how the brain's connectivity gives rise to individual differences in behavior and cognition.

The first genome-mapping efforts were fueled by technological innovations that dramatically increased feasible sequence length while lowering sequencing cost.[9] These same forces are likely to play a major role in shaping the future of connectomics. A broad spectrum of empirical strategies for mapping the connectome across a variety of species including humans is currently under development. New technologies enable the acquisition of progressively larger data sets with increasing resolution and accuracy. However, at the time of writing, it appears unlikely that a single empirical strategy for mapping the connectome will emerge. This has several reasons. First and foremost, the multiscale arrangement of neural elements and their connections demand that mapping techniques capture patterns that range over many orders of magnitude—no single technique may ever be optimal for capturing the network all at once. Every scale faces its own set of formidable technical challenges for collecting and analyzing connectome data, and promising new avenues are continually being developed. Relating connectome data to neural activity and behavior imposes additional requirements, such as collecting connectome maps in ways that are economical and preserve the integrity of the brain and the organism.

As a result, connectomics continues to evolve, utilizing an ever-increasing range of techniques for mapping structural brain connectivity. These techniques are beginning to deliver an abundance of data on brain connectivity in unprecedented detail, from the microscale of neurons to the macroscale of brain systems. In the next two chapters, we turn to a brief survey of some of the main empirical strategies that drive connectomics today.

4 The Connectome at the Microscale

The observation of individual neurons through a microscope or the rendering of fiber tracts of the human brain obtained from neuroimaging data represent two rather different approaches to mapping the connectome (figure 4.1). Microscopy directly visualizes the structure of individual neurons including their processes and synaptic connections, at varying degrees of spatial resolution in the micrometer to nanometer range. In contrast, neuroimaging relies on statistical inferences based on complex signals sampled from relatively large volumes of neural tissue on a scale of several millimeters. Currently, there are no noninvasive techniques for the direct visualization of individual cells and axons in the live human brain. Hence, there is a significant gap between micro- and macroscales. Techniques at the microscale allow the tracing and reconstruction of a small number of neural elements in exquisite detail but so far have fallen short of providing complete network diagrams (with the sole exception of *C. elegans*). Techniques at the macroscale can yield a global picture of a whole-brain network but do so at the expense of spatial resolution. Given this impasse, attaining the grand scientific objective of assembling a comprehensive map of the human connectome requires pursuing a combination of empirical strategies with complementary strengths and weaknesses. The next two chapters will introduce a broad range of techniques and approaches that are currently deployed in this endeavor, at the micro- and macroscale.

In the immediate future, significant progress in *human* connectomics will mainly derive from mapping connectivity among millimeter-scale volumes of neural tissue. In contrast, near-term prospects for acquiring comprehensive connectome maps of the human brain at cellular resolution are dim at best, as current methods face significant, though perhaps not insurmountable, obstacles and challenges. While the human connectome at microscale resolution may currently be beyond reach, cellular

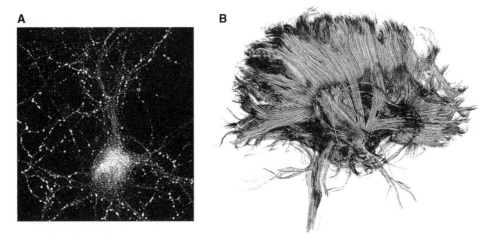

Figure 4.1
Microscopy and neuroimaging. (A) A fluorescence microscopy image of a cultured rat hippocampal neuron labeled for an abundant synaptic protein, synapsin, resulting in staining of numerous punctate synaptic sites. The image was taken by the author (modified after Sporns and Jenkinson, 1998). (B) A 3D computer reconstruction of callosal and cerebrospinal pathways obtained with diffusion magnetic resonance imaging. Courtesy of Martijn van den Heuvel (University Medical Center Utrecht, The Netherlands).

connectome maps of extended circuits or even of complete nervous systems of other animal species with smaller brains will soon become a reality. These studies will provide invaluable insights into the network architecture of microscopic and mesoscopic neural circuits that complement insights gained at the large scale from human neuroimaging. Since no single approach is able to provide a complete picture of the human connectome, integration among different connectome-mapping techniques is ultimately needed to harness their complementary strengths and mitigate their weaknesses.

In this chapter, we will survey some of the empirical approaches to mapping the connectome that are currently pursued at the microscale (see also Lichtman and Denk, 2011; Kleinfeld et al., 2011; Denk et al., 2012). While most strategies that rely on EM, LM, or tract tracing have not been applied to the mapping of human brain connectivity due to their invasive nature, they are included here because of their considerable power and promise for elucidating neural circuitry in model organisms, both vertebrate and invertebrate. Also, possible future application of EM or LM technology to postmortem human brain tissue may add to our understanding of the microcircuitry of the human brain.

EM Reconstruction of Neural Tissue

Arguably, of all strategies for mapping connectome networks, the reconstruction of cellular morphology and connectivity from EM data imaged at nanometer resolution offers the most complete and detailed information about the structure of neurons and the patterns of neural circuitry (Briggman and Bock, 2012). In principle, EM reconstructions allow the creation of a dense connectome map that includes all cells and synapses (including electrical junctions), possibly even with the inclusion of non-neuronal cells. In reality, the creation of such a map presents a formidable challenge, even for relatively small volumes of neural tissue. Braitenberg and Schüz (1998) estimated that 1 mm^3 of cortical gray matter of a mammalian brain contains more than 100,000 neurons, more than 700 million synapses, and more than 4 kilometers of axonal wiring.[1] Imaging of such a block of tissue at a typical EM resolution of $5 \times 5 \times 25$ nm would yield 1.6×10^{15} voxels, which translates into roughly 1.6 petabytes of raw data.[2] Making sense of such large amounts of data requires sound strategies for data compression and reduction.

All EM reconstruction approaches operate by assembling a three-dimensional (3D) description of fixed tissue on the basis of series of two-dimensional (2D) image stacks (figure 4.2, plate 2). Spatial resolution is often very high (on the order of a few nanometers) in the first two image dimensions, but in the third dimension resolution is limited by the section thickness (currently on the order of tens of nanometers). Because of this limitation, image stacks are composed of voxels with unequal dimensions, and various technical refinements are directed toward reducing this spatial anisotropy. Once image stacks have been acquired, a number of methodological challenges must be addressed, including the registration and alignment of multiple sections, the segmentation of imaged sections into discrete cellular objects, and the tracing of these objects through hundreds, and potentially thousands, of image slices. Virtually all past and current studies of neural architecture at the nanometer scale have relied either exclusively or in part on manual supervision and error correction by human experts, particularly for determining the continuity of neuronal objects through stacks of sections and for the detection of synapses between neurons. However, human intervention is extremely costly and time-consuming and thus cannot be pursued for reconstructions of larger tissue blocks or even whole nervous systems.[3] Thus, significant research efforts are directed toward achieving automation of the reconstruction pipeline, including the use of machine

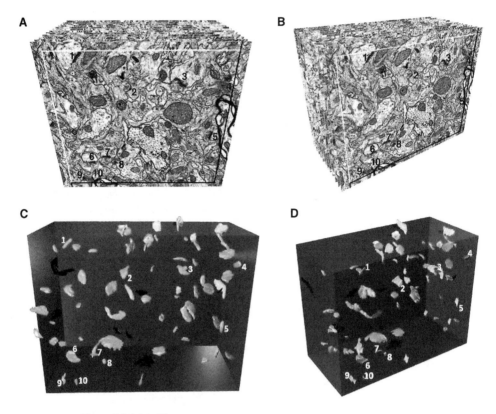

Figure 4.2 (plate 2)
Electron microscopy (EM) serial sectioning and reconstruction. Panels (A) and (B) show stacks of 12 EM serial sections, with each section covering an area of about 5 × 7 μm. The stack is rotated counterclockwise in the panels on the right, to provide a different visual perspective. Panels (C) and (D) show profiles of reconstructed synapses found within the volume; green objects represent asymmetrical synaptic profiles while red objects represent symmetrical synaptic profiles. Some of the synapses intersecting the front plane are labeled 1–10. Reproduced with permission from Merchán-Pérez et al. (2009).

learning techniques for automated segmentation and alignment of neural objects (e.g., Jain et al., 2010; Turaga et al., 2010; Jaume et al., 2011; Helmstaedter and Mitra, 2012) and the tracing of neuronal connections (Lu, 2011).

EM processing pipelines start with tissue preparation including fixation and labeling, followed by automated serial sectioning. The labeling step is important for improved detection of different cellular compartments—for example, cell membranes (surfaces) or synaptic junctions. A number of techniques for automated serial sectioning have been developed over the past few years. Serial block-face scanning EM (SBF-SEM; Denk and Horstmann, 2004) involves placing an ultramicrotome inside the imaging chamber of an electron microscope. A diamond knife removes thin slices from the fixed tissue block, and a scanning electron micrograph of the freshly cut block surface is taken. The process is repeated until the entire tissue block has been sectioned and imaged. Sectioning destroys the tissue block, and each sample can therefore be imaged only once. Successive removal of thin sections from a stationary tissue block improves alignment and distortion correction of adjacent images and thus aids in neuronal reconstruction. Mechanical removal of thin sections is not the only way to image neural tissue in three dimensions. Focused ion beam scanning EM (FIB-SEM; Knott et al., 2008) uses a nonmechanical approach to gradually ablate embedded tissue. Removal of tissue is effected by a focused beam of gallium ions which creates a milled surface that can be imaged with scanning EM. Removed tissue layers can be as thin as 15 nanometers, and the technique thus achieves very high spatial resolution in the depth dimension. A different approach is taken with a device called the automated tape-collection lathe ultramicrotome (ATLUM; Kasthuri et al., 2007). Automatically generated ultrathin sections are first collected on a carbon-coated tape, which is later processed for SEM imaging. Yet another alternative is the collection of serially sectioned material followed by transmission EM (ssTEM; Harris et al., 2006; Chklovski et al., 2010).

Regardless of how images of tissue sections are acquired, a necessary next step is to determine the locations and spatial arrangements of cellular objects (cells bodies, axons, synapses) with the ultimate goal of determining neuronal connectivity. Segmentation of EM images involves parsing of the image into distinct and internally coherent regions corresponding to individual cells or cellular compartments (figure 4.3). Full 3D reconstruction then faces the additional problem of determining the continuity of detected regions across multiple adjacent sections. Interestingly, some of the algorithms used to accomplish image segmentation are closely related to those employed in the regional parcellation of whole-brain imaging data acquired at the large scale (see chapter 5). Both problems involve the detection of coherent regions separated by boundaries in an imaged tissue section or on the cortical surface. The segmentation problem can in principle be tackled with two (mathematically equivalent) approaches, the detection and labeling of boundaries or the creation of an affinity graph between pixels that records whether two pixels belong to the same object or not (Jain et al., 2010).

Image	Boundary labeling	Segmentation

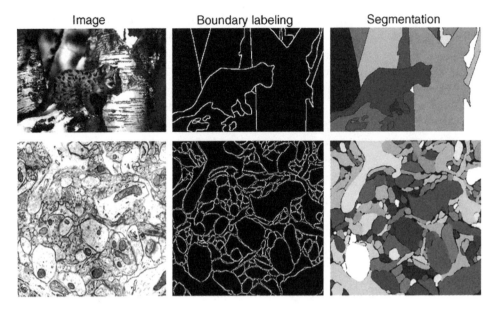

Figure 4.3
Image segmentation in electron microscopy (EM) connectomics. The left panel shows an example of a natural image (top) and a scanning EM image of mouse cortex (bottom). Boundaries between coherent image regions have been labeled in the center panels, and the segmented image regions are filled in (shaded in tones of gray) at the right. Modified (converted to grayscale) and reproduced with permission from Jain et al. (2010). See the original publication for more information on image sources.

Boundaries can be detected via image gradients by searching for sharp discontinuities in image properties such as intensity or texture, followed by error correction that capitalizes on contextual or global information to "clean up" boundaries that are inaccurate or incomplete. Once boundary detection is completed, individual voxels in an image are labeled as either belonging to a boundary or not. In contrast, the edges of affinity graphs link pairs of voxels (not necessarily adjacent in the image), and the sign of the edge indicates if the two voxels belong to the same or different regions. Hence boundaries exist between voxels, which increases spatial resolution. Affinity is determined on the basis of the similarity between voxels, again driven by image properties such as intensity or texture. Affinity graphs can be constructed not only for 2D images but also in 3D volumes linking voxels belonging to the same object across serial sections. Boundaries or affinity graphs can be expressed in binary form or, preserving the original similarity or dissimilarity measurements, in the form of probabilities.

A very large number of algorithms have been devised to solve various instances of the image segmentation problem. The specific qualities of EM images favor particular algorithms and processing parameters over others. Sebastian Seung and colleagues have argued that the most productive and efficient approach toward automated image segmentation in connectomics involves the use of machine learning to automatically select optimal algorithms (Jain et al., 2010). Human involvement, the main bottleneck in terms of speed and resources, will still be needed, particularly for the creation of training sets needed to optimize machine vision routines and for a final "merge and split" editing step to resolve inconsistencies. It is expected that more sophisticated use of contextual information, possibly across multiple spatial scales, will further increase the efficiency of automated segmentation routines.[4] Speed and accuracy of neurite reconstruction can be substantially improved by creating a skeletonized graph-like representation of fibers rather than retaining the full volume of contours (Helmstaedter et al., 2011) although the detection of synapses may still require full volume reconstruction. It should be noted that regardless of the level of precision of EM imaging or the accuracy of image registration, segmentation, and 3D linkage, some level of error in tracing and annotation will remain. Given the labor involved in manual error correction, statistical approaches are needed (Donohue and Ascoli, 2011). Helmstaedter et al. (2011) developed a statistical method for creating consensus estimates of neurite morphology from tracings performed by a large group of nonexpert individuals. This approach allows the identification of locations that are inconsistently captured and that need to be revisited and reexamined by experts. Despite the success of these refined reconstruction approaches, it seems likely that a certain level of error will remain and that statistical inference will eventually have to be performed on incomplete or noisy data. The extent to which this compromises the "ground truth" of synaptic connectivity is unknown.

Clearly, EM strategies for mapping the connectome are in rapid transition, and future technological developments will likely dramatically improve image resolution and automated 3D reconstruction. Current techniques have begun to reveal the cellular architecture of several neural structures in both vertebrate and invertebrate brains. Detailed analyses of small volumes of neural tissue in *Drosophila* (Cardona et al., 2010) and in rat hippocampus (Mishchenko et al., 2010) have demonstrated differences as well as similarities in cellular and subcellular organization of invertebrate and vertebrate neuropil. Reconstructions in

Drosophila revealed axonal cable lengths per tissue volume that were comparable to those found in vertebrates while the total length of dendritic processes was substantially greater. This increased profusion of dendrites was paralleled by a higher density of branch points. Synaptic density in *Drosophila* is relatively similar to that found in mammalian brains, but only when density is determined by counting presynaptic boutons. A much greater proportion of *Drosophila* synapses are found to be polyadic, that is, involve multiple postsynaptic sites for any single presynaptic site. Thus, the density of synaptic connections is significantly higher than that found in mammalian brains, where monadic synapses consisting of one presynaptic and one postsynaptic site prevail. Greater density of synaptic connections and dendritic branch points result in much greater compactness of microcircuits and in higher packing density of connection motifs.

Serial transmission electron microscopy was used to reconstruct neuronal circuitry in volumes of several hundred μm^3 of the rat hippocampus (Mishchenko et al., 2010). The study yielded important information about the density and size of neuronal compartments that can be used to discover or validate statistical rules of connectivity. For example, a long-standing statistical rule states that synapse formation between presynaptic boutons and postsynaptic dendrites is governed only by the spatial proximity of axons and dendrites (also called "Peters' Rule"; Braitenberg and Schüz, 1998). Contrary to the predictions of Peters' Rule, the EM data of Michchenko et al. (2010) indicated that synaptic density was only poorly predicted by the presence of axons near dendrites. Instead, dendritic circumference and ultrastructurally determined touches between dendritic spines and axons were strong predictors. Thus, synaptic connectivity cannot be inferred on the basis of axodendritic overlap alone, instead requiring the inclusion of parameters that depend on ultrastructural information.

This result implies that synaptic connectivity cannot be reliably inferred from geometric descriptions of cells and the overlap or relative proximity of their neurites—direct imaging of subcellular synaptic specializations like spines, presynaptic vesicles, or the postsynaptic density may be required. This endeavor may be aided by EM studies that include data on molecular distributions—for example, by visualizing synaptically expressed proteins. The inclusion of multiple molecular markers in a TEM analysis of a portion of the rabbit retina allowed the identification of cell types expressing different neurotransmitters as well as the mapping of complex connection motifs among different retinal cells (Anderson et al., 2011). The study confirmed the abundant existence of close spatial proximities between neurites that are not associated with synaptic contact, thus underscoring the necessity for ultrastructural mapping to derive network connectivity.

One of the most significant "next frontiers" in all connectome-mapping studies regardless of scale is the relationship between neuronal structure (morphology and connectivity) and function (dynamics and physiology). At the microscale, significant inroads have been made by combining physiological measurements and EM reconstruction carried out within the same tissue volume. Working in mouse primary visual cortex, Bock et al. (2011) first characterized functional properties of neurons such as their preferred stimulus orientation and then performed serial sectioning EM of the same tissue volume to determine synaptic interconnections and construct a network graph (figure 4.4, plate 3). The analysis of the connection diagram revealed convergence of inputs from multiple pyramidal cells with diverse orientation preference onto

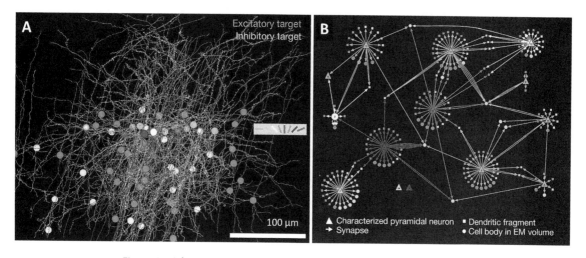

Figure 4.4 (plate 3)
Reconstruction and network diagram of physiologically identified neurons in mouse visual cortex. (A) The image shows a computer-generated, three-dimensional rendering of 14 functionally characterized visual neurons and their synaptic targets. Cell bodies, dendrites, and axons of the 14 neurons are colored according to their orientation preference. Target neurons are colored according to whether they are excitatory or inhibitory cells. (B) Directed graph of the anatomically reconstructed synaptic connections between the neurons shown in (A). Cell bodies of target neurons (excitatory, inhibitory) are shown as circles while other postsynaptic targets corresponding to dendritic fragments unconnected to cell bodies within the imaged volume are shown as squares. EM, electron microscopy. Modified and reproduced with permission from Bock et al. (2011).

inhibitory neurons. This pattern of convergence, while unrelated to the physiological specializations of the presynaptic cells, was partially predicted by axonal geometry, specifically the pairwise spatial overlap of their synaptic boutons. Another study that combined anatomy and physiology was carried out by Briggman et al. (2011) in the mouse retina (figure 4.5, plate 4). Following measurements of the physiological response properties of several hundred individual direction-selective ganglion cells, the tissue block containing their cell bodies, the adjoining inner plexiform layer, and part of the inner nuclear layer was fixed and subjected to SBF-SEM. Mapping of synaptic connections within a subnetwork of 24 starburst amacrine cells and 6 ganglion cells revealed highly nonrandom patterns of connectivity that form the structural substrate for previously observed asymmetries in physiological inputs of ganglion cells underlying their direction preference. Both studies (Bock et al., 2011; Briggman et al., 2011) present instructive examples of how physiological properties of cells can be traced to specific patterns of structural connections.

As this brief survey shows, the field of EM connectomics seems poised soon to deliver the first examples of connectivity matrices, at least from some restricted portions of the nervous system of a model organism. What is the potential of EM approaches for human connectomics? The difficulty of obtaining suitable material from either living or postmortem human brains will remain a major obstacle far into the future. All EM technology must operate on fixed specimens and involves the destruction of the brain in the process of acquiring images. This limits the potential of EM for revealing links between physiology and anatomy in the human brain. Nevertheless, EM has already begun and will continue to provide important information on the elementary rules that govern brain connectivity at cellular scales in both vertebrate and invertebrate nervous systems. It will be particularly important to determine the degree to which cellular connectivity is highly specific, varying from cell to cell in ways that matter for their functional specialization, or mainly random, implying that structural variation can be described in the form of parameters that characterize statistical distributions (see chapter 2). This question will also be addressed by complementary approaches that use light, not electron beams, to image cellular architecture.

Light Microscopy

Light microscopic (LM) approaches toward neuronal and circuit reconstruction face some of the same challenges encountered previously for

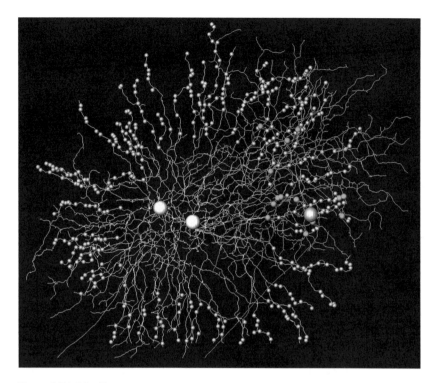

Figure 4.5 (plate 4)
Specificity of synaptic connectivity in the retina. The image shows the cell bodies (large round symbols) and dendrites of three neurons, one starburst amacrine cell (yellow) and two direction-selective ganglion cells (green), all reconstructed with SBF-SEM. Synaptic varicosities of the amacrine cell are marked by small yellow dots. Note that the dendrite of the amacrine cell shows substantial overlap with the dendrites of the two ganglion cells. However, the reconstruction reveals no synaptic connections between the amacrine cell and the ganglion cell at the left, while there are numerous synaptic connections between the amacrine cell and the ganglion cell at the right (magenta dots), demonstrating specificity of synaptic connections independent of dendritic overlap. The anatomical specificity of amacrine synapses is directly related to the physiological specificity (direction selectivity) of the ganglion cell. Courtesy of Kevin Briggman (Max-Planck-Institute for Medical Research, Heidelberg, Germany).

EM, including the need to correct for image distortions and deformations due to sectioning, to ensure accurate image alignment between sections, to segment images into neural objects, and to trace these objects across multiple sections while performing error correction. 3D neuronal reconstructions of neurons from LM images have a long history, with manual approaches increasingly supplanted by imaging algorithms. Digital and automated neuronal reconstruction techniques involve the tracing of axonal and dendritic processes and their translation into a geometric representation that can be used for quantitative comparison and modeling (Donohue and Ascoli, 2011). While LM reconstructions of individual cells have been carried out for some time, the determination of connectivity with the explicit goal of a network diagram or connection matrix has only just begun. LM has inherent limitations in this regard. With a resolution limit set by light diffraction at minimally 200 to 250 nm, LM approaches are generally considered to be insufficient for the unambiguous identification of small synaptic junctions, unmyelinated axons, dendritic spines, and other ultrastructural detail of neurons and neuronal processes. A new set of superresolution optical microscopy techniques aims at lowering the resolution limit by imaging individual fluorescently labeled molecules (Galbraith and Galbraith, 2011; Sigrist and Sabatini, 2012), but these approaches have yet to be applied to connectome studies.

Most LM approaches rely on various staining techniques to reveal the cellular morphology of neurons.[5] Sparse and monochrome stains include the Golgi method, as well as a host of tracers such as horseradish peroxidase, plant lectins, and lipophilic carbocyanine dyes used for visualizing long-range regional connectivity. These techniques allow the mapping of individual neuronal cell bodies and processes provided that there is sufficient separation and little overlap between imaged neurons. They, in general, do not permit the direct identification of synaptic contacts between cells—instead, neuronal connectivity must be inferred—for example, from the spatial overlap between axonal and dendritic processes of different cells. More recent technological developments involve the use of multiple colors to intracellularly label individual neurons within the same block of tissue (Livet et al., 2007). The expression of randomly varied combinations of green, yellow, cyan, and red fluorescent protein yields around 100 colors that can be individually distinguished and tracked (Lichtman et al., 2008). As is the case for all LM techniques, cellular details that are below the dimensions of the resolution limit cannot be imaged or mapped. A third set of techniques uses viral vectors—for example, herpes and pseudorabies virus—to reveal synaptic connectivity by utilizing the transsynaptic spread of virus particles from postsynaptic to presynaptic neurons. This technique allows for the joint identification of sets of pre- and postsynaptic neurons in sparsely labeled material.

In an earlier chapter (chapter 2) I discussed the influential idea that connection patterns among morphologically distinct classes of neurons in a given circuit may be described on the basis of empirically derived statistical patterns. These statistical descriptions deliver "canonical circuits," and candidates of such circuits have been proposed for cerebral cortex (Douglas and Martin, 2004). A comprehensive analysis of fully reconstructed individual neurons in cat visual cortex was carried out by Binzegger et al. (2004), resulting in a quantitative circuit diagram. Connections between neurons were not directly mapped but were inferred from the overlap of cell-type specific axonal and dendritic projection patterns. The resulting circuit topology (Binzegger et al., 2009; figure 4.6) exhibits high levels of connectivity among cell populations, with a few strong and many comparatively weak projections. If weaker projections are excluded, the circuit exhibits high clustering and a short path length, indicative of small-world organization. Dynamically, the circuit is stable, but the balance between excitatory and inhibitory influences places it close to the transition to dynamic instability. Canonical circuits that embody statistical rules of connectivity may become important ingredients for integrating specific details of microscale anatomy with large-scale connectivity.

Knife-edge scanning microscopy (KESM), developed by Yoonsuck Choe and colleagues (Mayerich et al., 2008; Choe et al., 2011; Chung et al., 2011; figure 4.7), allows the sectioning of whole animal brains while achieving near isotropic spatial resolution with voxel sizes below 1 μm. KESM has been successfully used for reconstructions of Golgi-stained neurons in the mouse brain. Using a similar technique, Li et al. (2010a) took a first step toward the construction of a cellular map of the whole mouse brain. A fixed and stained brain was sectioned at 1 μm thickness with an automatic micro-optical sectioning tomography (MOST) instrument and imaged with a light microscope. Data acquisition covered more than 15,000 coronal whole-brain sections, acquired over a period of more than 10 days and resulting in 8 terabytes of raw data. Sections reveal small brain structures including individual neurons and neuronal processes. The Golgi method stains only a random subset of all neurons and

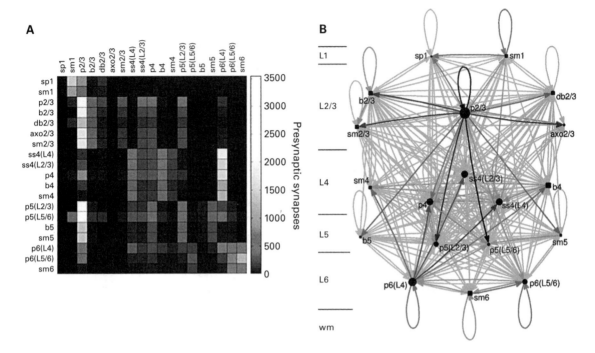

Figure 4.6
Network topology of a cortical canonical circuit. (A) Weighted and directed connection matrix between cell types of cat visual cortical area 17, with gray levels indicating the estimated number of synapses (target cell types are arranged as vertical columns). Abbreviations are as follows: b2/3, b4, b5 are basket cells in layer 2/3, 4, and 5, respectively; db2/3 are double bouquet cells in layer 2/3; p2/3, p4, p5, p6 are pyramidal cells in layer 2/3, 4, 5, and 6, respectively; ss4 are spiny stellate cells in layer 4; spiny stellate cells and pyramidal cells in layers 5 and 6 are further classified by their preferred layer of axonal innervations (e.g., L5/6). (B) The connection matrix as a directed graph, with the gray level of arrows indicating the number of synapses comprising the projection (black = maximal). Circles are excitatory cells, squares are inhibitory cells, and the symbol size is proportional to number of cells. Layers are numbered on the left; wm refers to white matter. Modified and reproduced with permission from Binzegger et al. (2009).

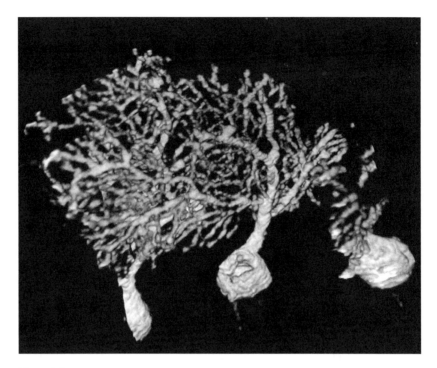

Figure 4.7
Purkinje cells reconstructed with knife-edge scanning microscopy. Cell bodies are at the bottom of the image, and dendrites extend upward. Courtesy of Yoonsuck Choe (Texas A&M University).

generally does not permit the identification of individual synapses. Therefore, MOST must infer synaptic connections based on the overlap of axonal and dendritic arbors and is thus not well suited for the dense reconstruction of a whole-brain connectome. Among the advantages of MOST are its applicability to the large scale of whole brain neural systems and its possible extension involving fluorescent labeling to further characterize neuronal phenotype.

The brain of the fruit fly *Drosophila melanogaster* contains about 100,000 neurons, most of which are found within a tiny volume easily fitting into a cube of around 500 μm on each side (Rein et al., 2002). Several efforts are under way to map the neural connectivity of *Drosophila* at the microscopic and mesoscopic scale. Yu et al. (2010) used genetic methods to divide a set of approximately 1,500 neurons that express a specific transcript related to courtship behavior into 100 distinct classes that are anatomically and functionally distinct. These 100 cell classes were placed into a 3D digital atlas, and their cellular polarity and presumptive connectivity pattern was determined, resulting in a network diagram that could be examined for sexual dimorphisms in the wiring pattern. Chiang et al. (2011) assembled a detailed and comprehensive connectivity map of the brain of *Drosophila* from high-resolution 3D images of approximately 16,000 single neurons. Each of these single neurons was positioned in and registered to one of two standard templates representing two adult (one male, one female) *Drosophila* brains. Anatomical segmentation of the neuropil stained for a synaptic marker protein yielded 58 morphologically distinguishable regions. In parallel, functional subdivision of the nervous system was performed by categorizing neurons into two classes: local interneurons and projection neurons. Processes of interneurons remain confined within a putative "local processing unit" (LPU) while processes of projection neurons connect LPUs to each other. Spatially distinct populations of local interneurons were taken to be a key criterion for the definition of LPU boundaries, and an analysis of the distribution of their cellular processes yielded 41 candidate LPUs which largely overlapped with anatomically segregated neuropil regions. Aggregation of processes extending between LPUs into a mesoscopic brain-wide wiring diagram resulted in a connection matrix, a weighted graph of LPUs linked by processes of projection neurons (figure 4.8, plate 5). Clustering of LPUs reveals distinct communities or modules, including four modules containing neurons primarily involved in vision, olfaction, audition, and locomotion. Clustering of neurons whose processes followed similar trajectories yielded 58 interregional fiber bundles or tracts, including 14 tracts that linked corresponding LPUs in the two hemispheres. While the study did not provide a complete cellular map and individually identified synaptic connections, it took a first important step toward characterizing the intermediate-scale (mesoscopic) arrangement of functionally coherent modules and processing elements in the fly brain. This mesoscopic description results from a subsampling strategy. Statistical analysis suggests that a sample of only a few thousand neurons is sufficient to provide an accurate representation of major cell groupings and their interconnections.

Color variations in the expression of transgenic fluorescent proteins (Brainbow; Livet et al., 2007) can densely label neuronal circuitry and thus offer one possible avenue toward tracing neurons and their connections for reconstructing dense connectomes (Lichtman et al., 2008). The application of this imaging strategy in complex 3D circuits is facing some difficulties related to the reliable and uniform expression of

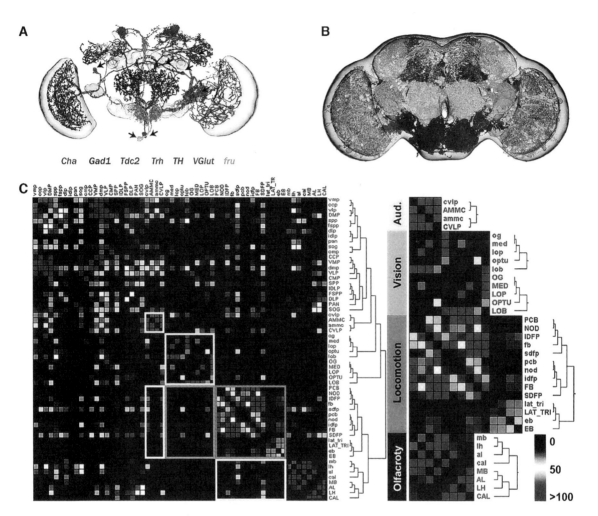

Figure 4.8 (plate 5)

Network diagram of the mesoscale *Drosophila* connectome. (A) Individual neurons were labeled using a fluorescent cell marker, imaged at high resolution and digitally mapped into standard brain coordinates. The image shows seven individually imaged neurons. (B) Composite image of cells colored by their membership in one of several dozen local processing units (LPUs). (C) Undirected network diagram summarizing inferred connections between LPUs. Prominent clusters corresponding to visual, auditory (Aud.), olfactory, and motor systems are reproduced at the right. For abbreviations of neural centers, please see original publication. Modified and reproduced with permission from Chiang et al. (2011).

marker proteins, the limited set of discriminable color variations (currently on the order of 100), and the limited resolution of LM fluorescent imaging. In a sparser environment, the technique has been successfully applied to tracing neuromuscular circuits in the mouse interscutularis muscle (Lu et al., 2009) and has revealed extensive individual variations and a spatial layout of neuronal processes that does not appear to minimize wiring length. Recent applications include zebrafish (Pan et al., 2011) and *Drosophila* (Hampel et al., 2011; Hadjieconomou et al., 2011).

Various genetic strategies for labeling neuronal structures including synapses allow fine temporal and spatial control and are thus good candidates for mapping connectivity profiles of specific cell types. One set of strategies relies on viruses which can be used for tracing monosynaptic connections because they afford both high transsynaptic specificity and signal amplification. A combination of viral vectors and transgenic strategies for targeting specific neuronal cell types allows for robust monosynaptic retrograde labeling of their input sources (Wickersham et al., 2007; Weible et al., 2010). While the approach enables the unambiguous detection of monosynaptic inputs to specific targets, the large number of cell types in the mammalian nervous system and the need to combine input maps from many different individual brains render the technique unsuitable for dense connectome-mapping efforts. It may be useful, however, for validation of EM reconstructions as well as for linking dense reconstructions obtained in smaller volumes to large-scale whole-brain maps of neuronal connections. Additional strategies for controlled labeling of specific synapses are available. One approach toward visualizing chemical synapses in specific neurons or neuronal populations involves a genetic method that combines high cellular specificity and temporally controlled expression (Li et al., 2010). Applied to cerebellar ganglion cells, the method generated new estimates of synaptic densities as well as new insights into synaptic distributions relative to other components of the cerebellar circuit.

Another approach to cellular reconstruction, array tomography, combines the advantages of immunofluorescence labeling with the high resolution of EM (Micheva and Smith, 2007; Micheva and Bruchez, 2012). Ultrathin serial sections cut from a fixed block of neural tissue can be repeatedly stained and imaged with different fluorescent markers, and the imaged sections can be processed further to yield EM micrographs and 3D volume reconstructions. Using this approach, targeting of a range of synaptically expressed proteins allows for the unambiguous identification of very large numbers of synapses in mouse cortex (Micheva et al., 2010).[6] The overlay of multiple layers of immunofluorescence, each labeling a different protein, yields colocalization patterns indicative of distinctive pre- and postsynaptic molecular components that define a repertoire of synaptic diversity.[7] The high-throughput capacity of array tomography opens an avenue toward creating a catalog of synaptic subtypes defined by their molecular composition across large regions of the brain. Such a catalog would be very useful for annotating connectome data recording patterns of connectivity with additional synaptic parameters.

The great utility of LM fluorescence imaging either alone or in combination with genetic protocols ensuring precise targeting of cell types complements the high resolution afforded by EM approaches. Additional challenges remain—for example, the detection of electrical junctions or the estimation of synaptic efficacy from morphological or molecular measurements. Factors that limit the usefulness of LM to human connectomics mirror those of EM techniques, including the invasiveness of the tissue preparation and the need for genetic modification in some LM approaches. Despite these limitations, efforts directed at the discovery of general rules that govern synaptic connectivity in the mammalian brain will ultimately prove fruitful for creating human connectome maps that span multiple scales. Perhaps most promising in this regard would be the combination of connectome maps of local circuits with those obtained from tract-tracing methods that specifically target long-range connections (see chapter 5), thus bridging cellular and large-scale connectome studies.

Statistics or Specificity?

The neuroanatomist Valentino Braitenberg once argued that the general shape of neurons is specified only in outline, with "details being filled in by largely random processes of growth." This randomness opened up the prospect of adopting statistical concepts to render the essential information contained in neuroanatomical structures, which according to Braitenberg was much preferable over "the very pessimistic note which the impossibility of unraveling precise circuitry for an enormous number of neurons would imply" (Braitenberg, 1990, p. 4). Braitenberg's pessimism expressed that it may be impossible to truly understand the bewildering intricacy of brain connectivity unless there is a discernable pattern, described by a set of statistical regularities. However, it is unclear whether such statistical regularities, assuming they can be identified, will be sufficient for a comprehensive description of the connectome. It seems that as more and more details of cellular morphology and connectivity are revealed, even minute structural variations, rather than representing "structural noise," are found to contribute to generating specific functionalities. One of the most important controversies in microscale connectomics centers on this conflict between specificity and randomness. The controversy plays out between proponents of statistical or population descriptions of circuitry (e.g., Douglas and Martin, 2011) and other investigators who point to the ever-increasing evidence for specificity in connections between individual neurons (e.g., Lee and Reid, 2011). If it turns out that specific patterns of connectivity cannot be reduced to statistical rules, the project of microscale connectomics and its integration with large-scale efforts will become significantly more difficult.

What should be included in a complete description of the human connectome at the microscale? Early efforts have put great emphasis on neurons and synaptic connections in the central nervous system (CNS). However, neurons can communicate, electrically and chemically, by other means, including gap junctions and extracellular signaling. In some tissues and circuits, gap junctions make up a large proportion of cellular communication, and the important role of gap junctions for electrophysiological processes is well documented. Slower and more diffuse biochemical signaling mechanisms by which cells can communicate include retrograde synaptic communication, neuromodulation, and hormonal control. Outside the CNS, a myriad of sensory and motor neurons innervate virtually all bodily tissues, relaying extremely important signals without which the integrity of the human body and adaptive behavior could not be maintained.[8] Neurons are chemically coupled to surrounding glial cells, particularly astrocytes, and the important roles of these nonneuronal cells for neuronal functioning are only beginning to be recognized (Fields, 2010). Finally, both neurons and glial cells interact with the brain's vasculature, and neurovascular coupling is important for energy metabolism and a key mechanism underlying noninvasive neuroimaging. Clearly, no microscale connectome can ever be fully comprehensive—even the most ambitious and fine-grained connectome efforts on the drawing boards today can only report on a small selection of cell types (mostly neurons), structures (mostly the CNS), and mechanisms (mostly synaptic).

Several orders of magnitude separate spines and dendritic branches from the myelinated tracts of the brain's white matter, to which we now turn. In moving to the meso- and macroscales of the brain, cellular resolution is lost. However, what is lost in resolution is gained in coverage, as modern histological and neuroimaging techniques can map the brain in its entirety and deliver complete descriptions of the connection topology at the large scale of regions and systems.

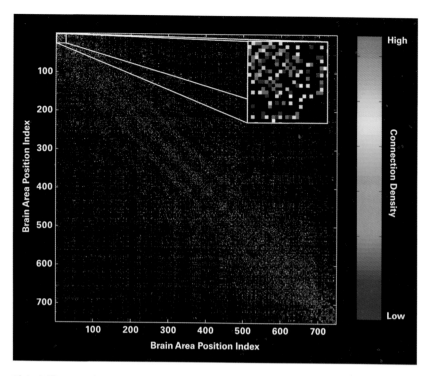

Plate 1 (figure 2.2)

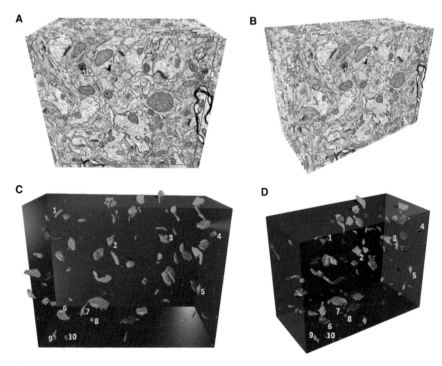

Plate 2 (figure 4.2)

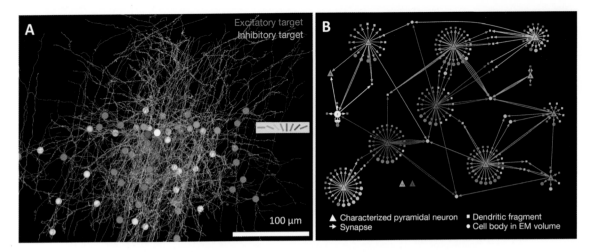

Plate 3 (figure 4.4)

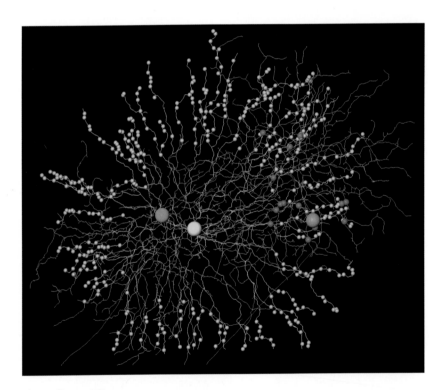

Plate 4 (figure 4.5)

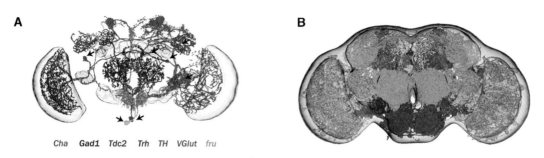

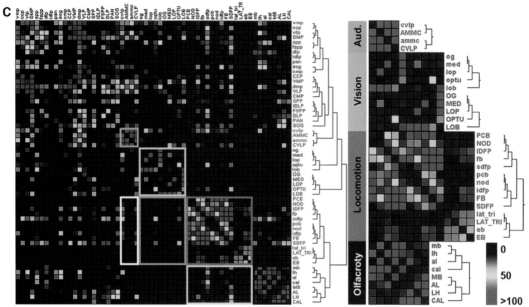

Plate 5 (figure 4.8)

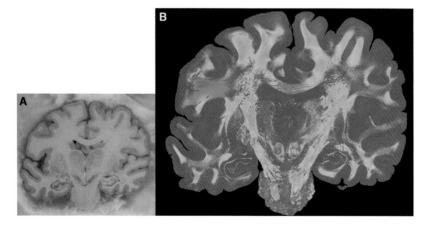

Plate 6 (figure 5.3)

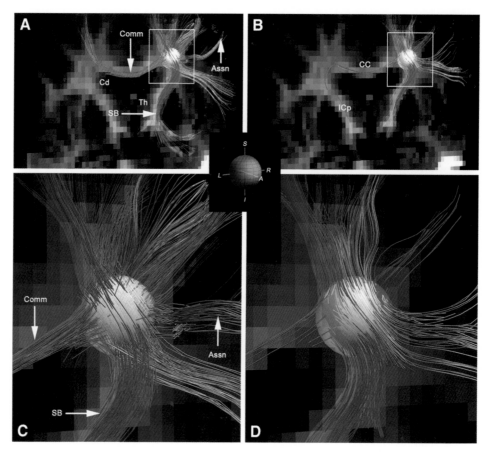

Plate 7 (figure 5.5)

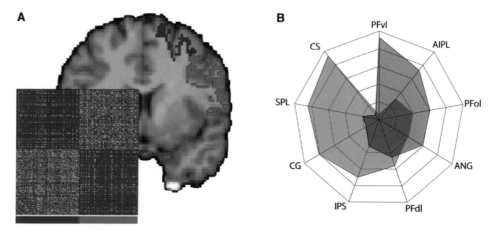

Plate 8 (figure 5.7)

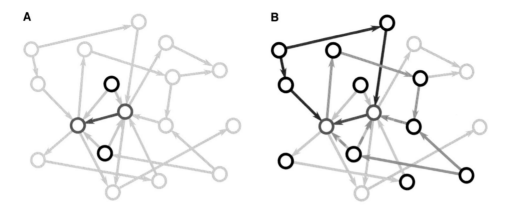

Plate 9 (figure 6.2)

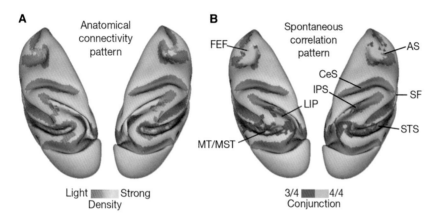

A
Anatomical
connectivity
pattern

Light ▓▓ Strong
Density

B
Spontaneous
correlation
pattern

FEF
MT/MST
LIP
IPS
CeS
AS
SF
STS

3/4 ▓▓ 4/4
Conjunction

Plate 10 (figure 6.3)

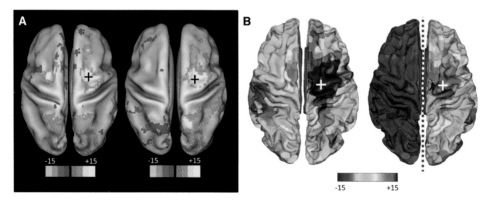

A
-15 +15   -15 +15

B
-15   +15

Plate 11 (figure 6.5)

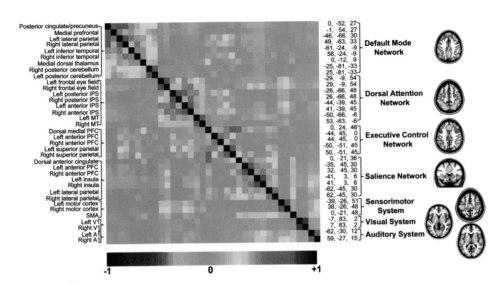

Plate 12 (figure 6.6)

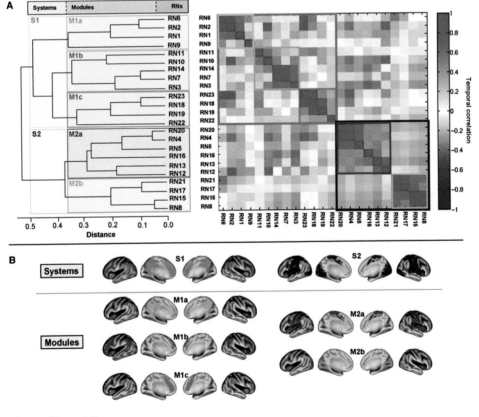

Plate 13 (figure 6.7)

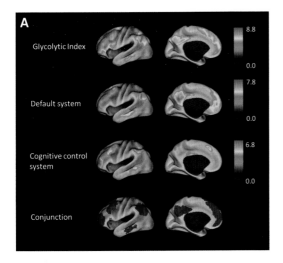

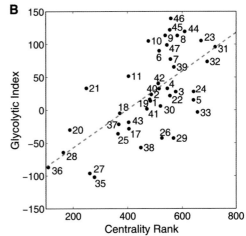

Plate 14 (figure 6.9)

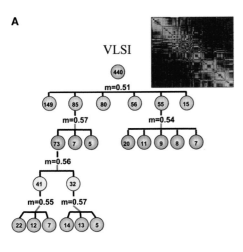

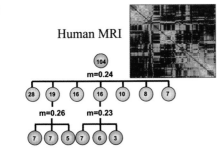

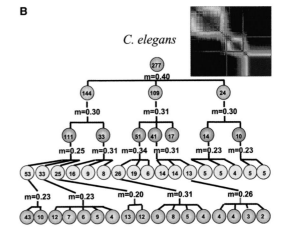

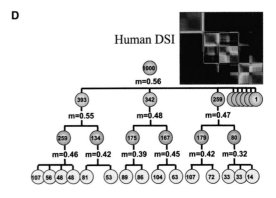

Plate 15 (figure 7.2)

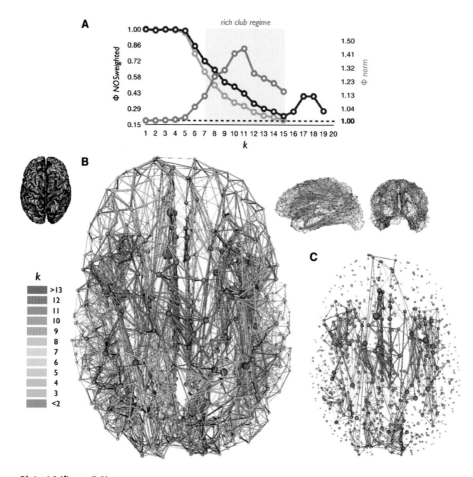

A

rich club regime

Φ NOSweighted

Φ norm

k

B

k

>13
12
11
10
9
8
7
6
5
4
3
<2

C

Plate 16 (figure 7.3)

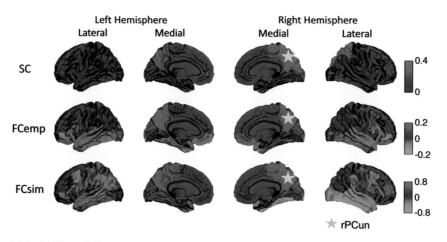

Left Hemisphere

Right Hemisphere

Lateral   Medial   Medial   Lateral

SC

0.4

0

FCemp

0.2
0
-0.2

FCsim

0.8
0
-0.8

★ rPCun

Plate 17 (figure 8.4)

5 The Connectome at the Macroscale

EM and LM techniques for dense connectome reconstruction currently operate within restricted (submillimeter) volumes of tissue and thus do not offer the field of view that would enable tracing of axons over longer distances. A different set of techniques is needed to accomplish this complementary goal. Mapping the human connectome at larger scales aims to deliver connectivity matrices of regions and interregional connections, most of which course through the brain's white matter. Charting the brain's major pathways has been an objective of classical neuroanatomy for over a hundred years, originally proceeding through a combination of anatomical dissection and histology (figure 5.1). The relation of these pathways to human cognition and its disturbances was a central concern for pioneers like the Viennese neurologist and psychiatrist Theodor Meynert, who began studying the projection fibers ("Projektionsfasern") of the brain 150 years ago.[1] Meynert became particularly interested in "cerebral architecture," major components of which were the "association systems" of fibers that linked brain regions both within and between hemispheres. Foreshadowing the core theme of connectomics, he wrote that "if we are acquainted with the principles upon which this mechanism [the brain] operates, we may infer its function from its structure, regarding the former as the natural outcome of the latter" (Meynert, 1885, p. 138). Almost in passing, when discussing the "arciform nerve-bundles" comprising the brain's white matter, Meynert notes that "the wealth of such fibres, and their variation in length, connecting as they do near and remote parts of the cortex, will suffice, without formulating an anatomical hypothesis, to unite any one part of the cortex to any other" (ibid., p. 150).

While commissural and association fibers of the brain have long been regarded as a plausible substrate for functional integration, creating a complete map of such connections for the human brain has been an

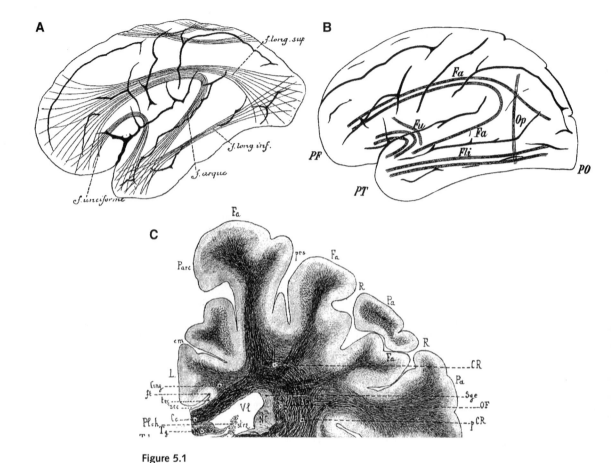

Figure 5.1
Nineteenth-century depictions of the brain's white matter architecture. (A) Diagram of major association pathways by Arthur Van Gehuchten (Van Gehuchten, 1894, p. 656). Pathways are f. long. sup., superior longitudinal fasciculus; f. long. inf., inferior longitudinal fasciculus; f. arque, arcuate fasciculus; f. unciforme, uniform fasciculus. (B) A similar illustration by Heinrich Obersteiner. In the accompanying text, Obersteiner described these pathways as designed "for bringing into *functional connection* distant parts of the brain and so providing the mechanism for concerted actions" (Obersteiner, 1890, pp. 348–349; italics mine). PF, frontal pole; PT, temporal pole; PO, occipital pole; Fa, fasciculus arcuatus; Fu, fasciculus uncinatus; Fli, fasciculus longitudinalis inferior; Op, fasciculus occipitalis perpendicularis. (C) A drawing of the superior and inferior segments of the corona radiata (CR), stained using the method of Weigert and drawn by M. Gillet, from the monumental *Anatomie des Centres Nerveux* by Jules Dejerine (Dejerine, 1895, p. 10). Note the intricate texture of stained association, commissural and projection fibers.

elusive goal. In part, this was due to the extreme delicacy of nervous tissue, subject to rapid decay after death, and the lack of sensitive and reliable empirical methods for tracking connections over long distances through the brain's volume. Today, new methods for charting neuroanatomical connections invasively with chemical tracers or noninvasively with methods from neuroimaging have become available. At present, these methods are deployed in several concerted efforts to compile whole-brain maps of structural connectivity with the explicit aim of creating network descriptions of brain architecture.

Tract Tracing

Tract tracing represents a set of anatomical mapping strategies that rely on the sparse labeling of cells with a tracer substance to visualize their projections throughout the brain (Kötter, 2007). Different anterograde and retrograde tracers, injected intracellulary or applied extracellularly, have been used over several decades in numerous anatomical studies of neuronal projections in various mammalian nervous systems. Tract-tracing studies formed the basis of some of the very first large-scale connection matrices, collected for the corticocortical projections of the cat (Scannell et al., 1995, 1999) and macaque monkey (Felleman and Van Essen, 1991), and the first examples of neuroinformatics databases specifically designed for collating information on brain connectivity (e.g., "Collations of Connectivity Data on the Macaque Brain," or CoCoMac; see Kötter, 2004). Tract tracing is usually best suited for long-range interregional projections since it cannot resolve circuitry in the immediate vicinity of the tracer injection site. By their nature, anatomical tract-tracing methods are highly invasive, requiring tracer injection, fixation, and histological processing of brain sections. Furthermore, the assembly of a comprehensive connectome map necessarily involves the combination of data from many individuals and tracer injections into numerous anatomical sites. These limitations preclude studies of large populations of individuals as well as the systematic assessment of individual differences or longitudinal changes across time. However, unlike diffusion imaging, the technique allows the direct quantification of axonal fibers, including their directionality and branching patterns, at microscopic resolution, and it sensitively detects both strong and weak pathways.

Virtually no tract-tracing data are available for the human brain, and progress in the development of postmortem axonal tracing methods suitable for the human brain has been slow. However, tract tracing remains important in other mammalian species, including in nonhuman primates, not least of all for its role in providing essential validation for other noninvasive large-scale mapping strategies such as diffusion MRI (see below). Most previous studies of anatomical pathways have reported their presence or absence or have recorded their strength on an ordinal (strong, intermediate, weak) scale. Increasingly, anatomical tracing is accompanied by the application of sophisticated quantitative methods for establishing precise estimates for the magnitude or density of individual projections.

Two recent examples involve tracing of structural connections in mouse and macaque monkey. Wang et al. (2011b) carried out a detailed mapping study of corticocortical connections of two central areas of mouse visual cortex, the lateromedial field and the anterolateral field, both recipients of major projections from area V1. Injections of an anterograde tracer were used to quantify the density of synaptic boutons in each projection pathway. Labeling patterns revealed characteristic differences in the density of projections to the lateromedial field and anterolateral field. These differences support the idea that mouse visual cortex is organized into two parallel visual processing streams analogous to the ventral and dorsal streams of primate visual cortex (Wang et al., 2012). Importantly, differences in the projections of the lateromedial field and anterolateral field only emerged if projection densities were taken into account—a binary representation recording the presence of absence of projections would have revealed no differences as both areas project to a common set of target regions.

Significant variations in the density of corticocortical pathways, consistent across individuals, were reported recently for new tract-tracing data collected in the macaque monkey (Markov et al., 2011). The weight of interregional connections was estimated by measuring the "fraction of labeled neurons" detected after injection of a retrograde tracer into a target region. Quantitative analysis revealed a remarkable range of connection weights spanning over five orders of magnitude and scaling according to a lognormal distribution (figure 5.2), including a significant number of previously unreported pathways. The study confirmed earlier results indicating a robust relationship between metric connection distance and connection density, with a strong bias in density towards local and short interregional projections. The data reported in Markov et al. (2011) and Wang et al. (2011b) strongly suggest that functional specialization of cortical regions not only depends on the presence or absence of connections but relies on their differential density or weight. These

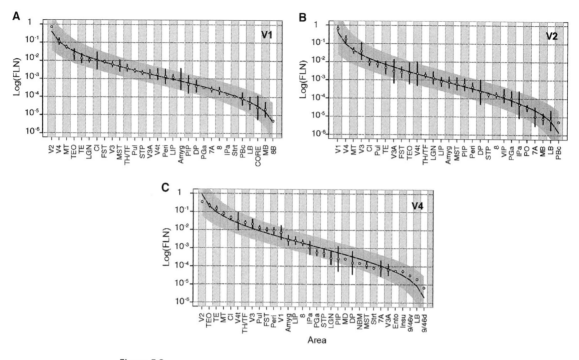

Figure 5.2
Density profiles for interregional connections of macaque visual regions. Connection density is measured as the "fraction of labeled neurons" (FLN) measured after injection of retrograde tracers into three target regions, visual regions V1 (A), V2 (B), and V4 (C). The plots show log-transformed and rank-ordered connection densities from a set of cortical and subcortical regions, averaged over several injections. The fitted curve represents a log-normal distribution. Note that connection density varies over at least 5 orders of magnitude, with an overall log-normal shape that is shared between the three regions. Note also that each region's connection profile is unique. More recently, quite similar results were obtained for projections in mouse cortex (Wang et al., 2012). For abbreviations, please consult the original publication. Modified and reproduced with permission from Markov et al. (2011).

findings underscore the need to develop reliable and validated measures that can estimate the magnitude of projections in large-scale neuro-anatomy, regardless of the technique employed.

Several coordinated efforts are under way to compile connectome data at the mesoscale. A large group of investigators (Bohland et al., 2009) proposed an effort to assemble a connectivity matrix for the mouse brain by using standard tract-tracing protocols but scaling up the project to achieve uniform whole-brain coverage and quantitative analysis. In the spirit of the proposal, the Brain Architecture Project (http://brainarchitecture.org) aims at developing standardized high-throughput methodologies for mapping whole-brain structural connectivity in model organisms at the mesoscale, as well as devising new techniques for mapping structural connections in postmortem human brain. The Mouse Connectome Project (http://www.mouseconnectome.org), centered at the University of California, Los Angeles, aims to provide a 3D whole-brain connectome atlas by combining data from approximately 400 injections of anterograde and retrograde tracers. These injections will be applied to a grid of positions, and projection patterns will be registered to a 3D standard reference atlas. A similar project is currently under way at the Allen Institute for Brain Science. Thus, the prospects for a achieving a mesoscale mouse connectome within the very near future appear bright.[2] Such a connectome would likely comprise several hundred anatomically distinct neural regions and their mutual directed projections.

Chemical tracers combine high sensitivity with the ability to map whole-brain circuitry, but they cannot be used in humans. 3D polarized light imaging (3D-PLI) offers a new approach to large-scale connectomics that can be applied to postmortem human brain and allows the tracing of axonal fiber bundles at a resolution of hundreds of micrometers (Palm et al., 2010; Axer et al., 2011). The technique exploits optical properties of thin sections of brain tissue, specifically due to the interaction of polarized light with the spatially anisotropic fiber architecture of the brain's white matter (figure 5.3, plate 6). Collection of polarized light images at different polarization angles and acquired from thin (100-μm) sections of fixed whole brain is followed by computational reconstruction of 3D fiber models at each voxel. The pathways of long-range projections can then be reconstructed using various tractography techniques (covered in more detail in the next section). This opens the possibility that 3D-PLI might be used in the near future for compiling a comprehensive description of fiber architecture in the human brain at a spatial resolution that is superior to that offered in current diffusion MR technology. Such a description would be very useful for validating tracts derived from noninvasive imaging data. 3D-PLI shares some of the limitations of tract tracing as it relies on the availability of postmortem brains and does not allow for longitudinal or population studies.

Tract tracing serves an important role in connectomics, as it joins the microscales tackled by EM and LM approaches to the macroscale of whole-brain anatomy. EM (and, to some extent, LM) deliver connectional information with high specificity. In contrast, the profusion of

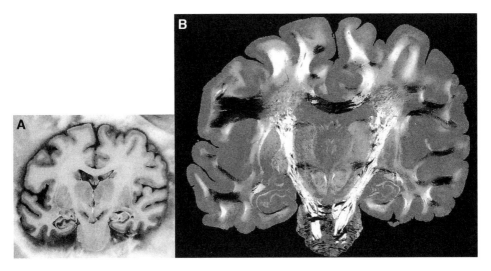

Figure 5.3 (plate 6)
Three-dimensional polarized light imaging (3D-PLI) of a human brain. After removal and
fixation, the brain was embedded in gelatin and frozen, followed by sectioning in the
coronal plane on a cryostat microtome with a section thickness of 100 μm. (A) Blockface
image of a representative section, clearly showing gray and white matter regions. (B) After
imaging of the section in polarized light and various transformations to extract information
about the orientation of fibers, 3D fiber vectors can be graphically visualized. The color
map encodes the direction of fibers at each position: left–right (red), basal–dorsal (up–
down, green), and rostral–occipital (in–out, blue). Modified and reproduced with permission from Palm et al. (2010).

axonal processes labeled by even small injections of tracer compounds
generally rules out precise tracking of individual axons, nor does it
allow the unambiguous identification of synaptic junctions between
individual cells. Tract-tracing data are inherently statistical in nature,
reporting connection densities and distributions while leaving the
issue of connection specificity unresolved. However, while tract-tracing
approaches are well suited for detecting long-range axonal projections,
it appears doubtful that dense reconstructions at the EM level can be
scaled up to cover distances of many millimeters or centimeters in the
foreseeable future. Tracking individual axons over a modest distance of
1 cm requires error-free reconstruction across an image stack of nearly
half a million slices (assuming 25-nm section thickness). The strengths
and weaknesses of dense EM reconstructions, other related LM strategies, and of tract tracing appear largely complementary, and given this
methodological trade-off, a feasible near-term goal may be to compile an integrated statistical description of local and long-range brain

connectivity drawing on EM, LM, and tract tracing in a model organism like the mouse.

We now turn to the status and promise of compiling a map of the human connectome from data about structural connectivity acquired with modern MRI methods. Most of the following discussion will focus on parcellation and structural connectivity of the human cerebral cortex. This bias reflects the challenges that are involved in establishing objective regional partitions and validated interregional connections for this large subdivision of the brain. It should be emphasized that all methods discussed in the remainder of the chapter fully extend to subcortical structures and that these structures are naturally included in all ongoing and future efforts to map the human connectome.

Magnetic Resonance Connectomics

There are two main avenues toward collecting data on structural connections in the human brain with magnetic resonance (MR) technology. Before turning to a set of techniques that are of central interest for mapping the connectome in individual human brains, we briefly discuss a more indirect approach based on brain morphometry. The method infers the presence of structural connections on the basis of cross-correlations in cortical thickness (Lerch et al., 2006). The morphometric assessment of cortical thickness is carried out on MR images that are segmented into cortical gray and white matter, and measurements for each pair of vertices or regions on the cortical surface are then cross-correlated across individuals in a population. Validation studies have shown that the resultant correlation maps resemble pathways known from classical neuroanatomy or mapped with diffusion MRI (Lerch et al., 2006). The neurobiological mechanisms that drive these cross-correlations are only partially understood and probably involve developmental mechanisms in addition to adult neuroplasticity. Because correlations in cortical thickness are estimated across a population of multiple brains, the approach cannot be used for measuring structural connectivity in individual participants. Nevertheless, the approach was instrumental for creating some of the very first connectome maps at the large scale (He et al., 2007) and, in combination with network analysis, continues to be deployed in clinical and developmental contexts (Bernhardt et al., 2011; Chen et al., 2011).

The other main branch of MR connectomics involves the mapping of structural connectivity based on diffusion MRI and tractography (Basser et al., 1994; Le Bihan et al., 2001; Le Bihan, 2003; Johansen-Berg and Behrens, 2009; Hagmann et al., 2010a; Behrens and Sporns, 2012; Van Essen and Ugurbil, 2012). Diffusion MRI is based on measurements of the diffusion anisotropy of water or other small molecules within biological tissue, and the technique is widely applied in the noninvasive study of skeletal and heart muscle as well as the brain. Diffusion anisotropy arises as a spatial asymmetry of the random displacement of water molecules undergoing Brownian motion (figure 5.4). The asymmetry is due to the presence of oriented cellular structures which restrict and amplify diffusion in specific directions. In the case of the brain, these cellular structures might correspond to myelin sheaths surrounding axonal processes. Measuring diffusion anisotropy thus provides information on the spatial orientation of myelinated axon bundles coursing through the brain's white matter. Diffusion signals can be detected in an MR scanner, exploiting a relationship between the diffusion-related displacement probability density function and the observed MR signal. Appropriate sampling of the MR signal by using motion-sensitized magnetic gradients oriented in multiple directions allows the recovery of the diffusion signal at each voxel. Sampling a larger number of diffusion directions generally improves resolution, which is important for voxels that contain crossing fibers (see below), but it also tends to increase imaging time. As is the case with all MR imaging modalities, signals are subject to a host of noise sources, from scanner instability to eddy currents and physiologically induced artifacts. In the latter category, uncontrolled tissue movements in conjunction with physiological processes such as cardiac pulsation and respiration can introduce unwanted signal components (Chung et al., 2010; Walker et al., 2010).

It is important to emphasize that diffusion imaging and tractography cannot directly trace or visualize anatomical connections. Rather, the approach rests on the inference of a connectivity model that best explains an observed MR signal distribution.[3] The original approach, diffusion tensor imaging, assumed that each voxel can be characterized by a single diffusion direction, corresponding to a single coherent axonal bundle. However, voxels may contain crossing fibers that belong to different axonal tracts originating and terminating in widely dispersed regions of the brain. Such crossing fibers can give rise to a complex diffusion signal that is no longer adequately modeled by a simple diffusion tensor but constitutes a mixture of diffusion directions. Complex fiber architecture is encountered in numerous regions of white matter, possibly comprising a majority of all white matter voxels. Several methods for imaging

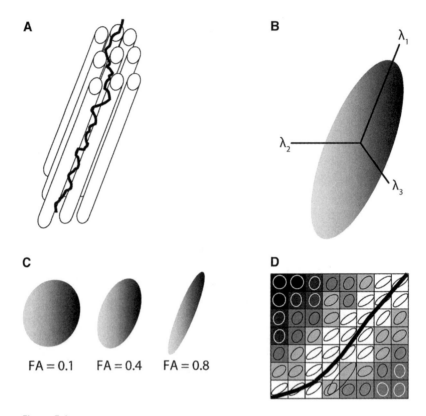

Figure 5.4
Diffusion MRI and tractography. (A) A schematic diagram showing the diffusion of a water molecule (along the black line) in a tissue volume that contains oriented fibers. Diffusion is restricted in any direction that is perpendicular to the orientation of the fiber bundle. (B) At each voxel the diffusion of water can be expressed as a tensor defined by three principal eigenvectors (shown here as arrows) and their associated eigenvalues ($\lambda 1, \lambda 2, \lambda 3$). (C) The tensor model describes the principal direction of diffusion and the degree of fractional anisotropy (FA), which can range between 0 (no anisotropy) and 1. (D) Multiple tensors form a tensor field, and streamline tractography proceeds by tracing a line through the field, corresponding to the trajectory of a putative axonal fiber. Multiple streamlines can be seeded throughout the white matter, and their trajectories can be combined across the brain (see, e.g., figure 4.1B). Reproduced with permission from Johansen-Berg and Rushworth (2009).

complex fiber architecture aimed at resolving multiple diffusion directions at single voxels have been proposed (e.g., Behrens et al., 2003; Tuch et al., 2003). One such approach is diffusion spectrum imaging (DSI), which measures the full 3D distribution of the displacement probability density function (Wedeen et al., 2005). Figure 5.5 (plate 7) shows an application of DSI to the centrum semiovale, a white matter region that is notoriously difficult to resolve. Located underneath frontoparietal regions of cortex, multiple pathways intersect in this region including callosal fibers traveling mediolaterally, long association fibers extending rostrocaudally, and fibers running in the corona radiata (cf. figure 5.1). Comparative analyses indicate that these major pathways are jointly detected by DSI in concordance with known neuroanatomical patterns of connectivity (Wedeen et al., 2008).

Most tractography algorithms can be classified as either deterministic or probabilistic. Deterministic algorithms construct individual "streamlines" corresponding to putative axonal fibers by local path integration along principal diffusion directions (Conturo et al., 1999; Mori et al., 1999). Deterministic tractography can be adapted to handle fiber crossings and take into account complex distributions of diffusion directions within single voxels (Wedeen et al., 2008). Multiple tractography streamlines obtained by propagating fibers from a large number of seed locations in the white matter can be combined into pathways that link pairs of gray matter voxels or regions (Hagmann, 2005; Hagmann et al., 2007). In contrast to deterministic tractography, which only records connections between voxels or regions for which at least one streamline has been found, probabilistic tractography estimates connection probabilities between all voxel or region pairs (Behrens et al., 2003, 2007). Probabilistic approaches deliver information about the uncertainty of each connection given the data, information that is fundamentally lacking from representations based on deterministic streamlines.

To date, most deterministic or probabilistic tractography algorithms operate primarily on local diffusion estimates but do not take into account more global constraints on brain connectivity such as conservation of tissue volume or additional local measures that report on tissue microstructure. One example of the application of global constraints involves an optimization algorithm for creating connectome maps that searches for connectivity patterns that fit both diffusion data and tissue volume constraints (Sherbondy et al., 2009). Other approaches aim at combining global tractography and local measurement of connectional microstructure into a single algorithmic framework (Sherbondy et al.,

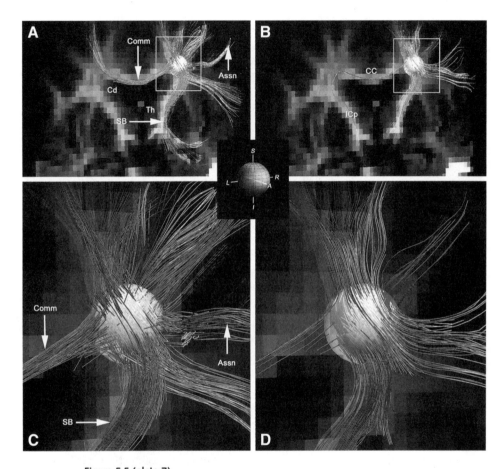

Figure 5.5 (plate 7)
Diffusion imaging of intersecting fibers. The four panels show fibers reconstructed with streamline tractography within the centrum semiovale. Panels A and C show results from diffusion spectrum imaging (DSI) while panels B and D show results obtained with diffusion tensor imaging (DTI). Multiple fiber pathways intersect in the area marked by a white sphere: Commissural (Comm) fibers traveling through the corpus callosum (CC) are shown in red/orange; long association (Assn) fibers are shown in green; corona radiate fibers are shown in blue. Note the great reduction and spurious trajectories of intersecting tracts in DTI scans. Cd, caudate nucleus; ICp, posterior limb of internal capsule; SB, subcortical bundle projection fibers; Th, thalamus. Reproduced with permission from Wedeen et al. (2008).

2010). Based on the assumption that microstructural characteristics such as axon diameter (see below) remain constant along the entire length of a pathway, tractography and microstructure estimates can be jointly optimized to fit the observed signal distribution.

The end result of whole-brain tractography can be summarized in a connection matrix recording estimates of the magnitude or strengths of long-range interregional connections. For data obtained with deterministic tractography, the number and density of streamlines connecting voxels or regions is often taken as an indication of the magnitude of the pathway. If streamlines are aggregated between anatomical parcels of unequal size or volume, estimates of the "strength" or magnitude of structural connectivity are often expressed as a streamline density, derived by dividing off the combined volumes of the connected parcels (e.g., Hagmann et al., 2007, 2008).[4] Probabilistic tractography delivers estimates for the likelihood of projections, which generally differ depending on the direction in which tractography is carried out. These asymmetrical probabilities must be transformed into (undirected) projection magnitudes or densities. It remains unclear how streamline counts, densities, or connection probabilities translate to the morphology of the underlying biological substrate (Jbabdi and Johansen-Berg, 2011), and joint imaging and histological work directed at clarifying these relations are urgently needed.

Once tractography is complete, unless further steps are taken to partition the brain into anatomically or functionally defined regions (see the next section), the result is a connectivity map for individual voxels (usually comprising all gray matter regions of the brain) or, in the case of the cerebral cortex, for individual vertices forming a surface mesh. This high-resolution connectome map reports connectivity among many thousands of nodes representing individual surface or volume elements at a scale of several millimeters. The locations and boundaries of these nodes result from an essentially random process of dividing the brain into small volume elements during image acquisition. These nodes therefore do not represent neurobiologically distinct subdivisions or functionally defined units. Network analysis can be performed on these high-resolution partitions or on more compact connectome maps whose nodes and edges correspond to coherent functional elements defined on the basis of neurobiological criteria (see the next section).

Diffusion imaging and tractography are subject to a number of methodological biases and limitations. Diffusion imaging only works in parts of the brain where diffusion is anisotropic—for example, cerebral white matter. For the most part, this excludes gray matter voxels and thus prevents the detection of connections in gray matter or in unmyelinated axons in general. Because of the nature of molecular diffusion, the method currently cannot provide any information about the direction of axonal pathways, nor can it reveal axonal branching. Shallow fiber crossings which result in closely spaced diffusion maxima are difficult to distinguish from cases where fibers converge and diverge without crossing (so-called "kissing" fibers). Fiber-tracking algorithms tend to be biased towards the detection of shorter fiber tracts involving fewer reconstruction steps. Weaker tracts can be difficult to identify in the presence of much stronger pathways as their diffusion signals become harder to detect. Finally, statistical approaches towards resolving complex fiber architecture rest on various assumptions about how the diffusion signal is generated and measured. Intensive efforts are under way to address these biases and limitations, to validate existing diffusion MR technology against other methods that measure anatomical connectivity more directly, and to obtain additional information from the imaging signal that can further characterize structural brain connectivity.

Diffusion MRI not only delivers information about fiber orientation that can be used for tractography. The fractional anisotropy (FA) expresses the degree to which a voxel's diffusion profile deviates from being equal in all directions (see figure 5.4). FA is thought to depend on a combination of several microstructural features such as the diameter of fibers, their local density, and the degree to which they are myelinated. Together with other related measures of diffusion, the FA can provide an indication of white matter "integrity"—for example, the local coherence of axonal fibers or their myelination status. Characteristic changes in FA are observed during brain development, and in the adult brain FA can index structural alterations due to neuroplasticity (see chapter 3). More recent studies have shown that diffusion MRI can also disclose other important microstructural parameters such as the local distribution of axonal diameters and the density of axons within imaged white matter voxels (Alexander et al., 2010). Zhang et al. (2011) proposed an improved detection scheme for the robust estimation of axonal diameters even in places where the orientations of diffusion directions are dispersed. Axonal diameter is an important structural parameter because it may be related to the axon's speed of transmission and thus the conduction delay between brain regions, as well as the rate at which the axon transmits information (Perge et al., 2012). Currently, there are no noninvasive ways to assess the physiological efficacy of a structural connection. Some studies have used the myelination status of tracts as a proxy for connectional efficacy, estimated from FA or the mean diffusivity (e.g., Hagmann et al., 2010b) or from the level of macromolecules including myelin (van den Heuvel et al., 2010). However, these measures only capture some aspects of the microstructural or molecular organization of fiber anatomy and do not record biophysical parameters that contribute to synaptic strength or efficacy.

Given the nature of diffusion imaging and tractography, it is important to validate results obtained from these approaches with more direct observations of connectivity obtained through anatomical methods. One avenue involves the comparison of axonal tracts reconstructed from diffusion imaging and tractography carried out in postmortem human brain with subsequent anatomical dissection, a technique that has recently become feasible (Miller et al., 2011) and should soon allow progress in this direction. Another avenue towards validating data from noninvasive imaging is the use of animal models where invasive anatomical approaches are possible, particularly nonhuman primates.[5] In macaque monkey, Schmahmann et al. (2007; see also Dauguet et al., 2007) compared observations on several long association fiber bundles obtained by diffusion imaging with results from autoradiographic tract tracing, a sensitive method for tracing long-range connections in histological material. Comparisons of the two techniques showed good overall agreement, thus supporting the notion that diffusion imaging can indeed map anatomically verifiable fiber tracts in humans (figure 5.6). While these initial studies are encouraging, agreement or disagreement is largely established on the basis of visual comparison. More detailed analyses should include quantitative comparison of connectivity matrices and metrics of network topology (e.g., Hagmann et al., 2008).

MR technology, and particularly diffusion imaging, stands out among other strategies for mapping the human connectome. It alone permits the assembly of connectivity maps in a manner that is noninvasive and relatively economical. Continued technological innovation—for example, the development of new pulse sequences that greatly accelerate acquisition times (Feinberg et al., 2010)—helps to improve both signal quality and ease of application. Diffusion imaging allows studies of large human populations and the longitudinal assessment of change and plasticity across the human life span from early development into senescence. Other distinct advantages are its applicability to individual whole brains, without the need to compose connection maps assembled from multiple individuals and reported in a standard reference frame. At this time, all

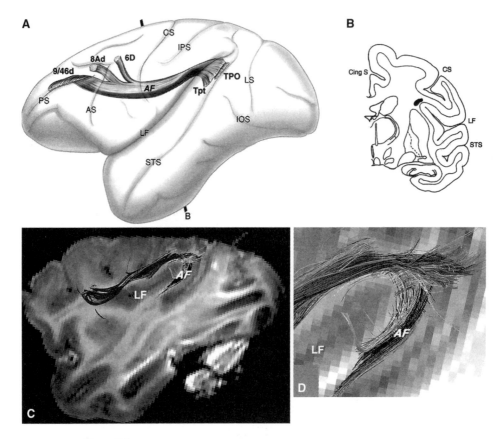

Figure 5.6
Comparison of diffusion imaging/tractography and monkey tract-tracing data. Panels A
and B show results obtained from tract tracing using an autoradiography labeling technique. Panels C and D show reconstructed fiber tracts after imaging of macaque cortex
with DSI. The figure depicts the arcuate fasciculus (AF). Cortical landmarks: AS, arcuate
sulcus; CS, central sulcus; IPS, intraparietal sulcus; IOS, inferior occipital sulcus; LF, lateral
fissure; LS, lateral sulcus; PS, principal sulcus; STS, superior temporal sulcus; Cing S, cingulate sulcus. Cortical regions: 6D, frontal area 6D; 8Ad; dorsal frontal area 8A; 9/46d, dorsal
prefrontal area 9/46; TPO; area TPO of the superior temporal sulcus; Tpt, superior temporal
area Tpt. Modified (converted to grayscale) and reproduced with permission from Schmahmann et al. (2007).

EM and most LM strategies operate only on fixed (ex vivo or postmortem) specimens that are destroyed during serial sectioning and imaging. Some strategies, in addition, need the insertion of genetic markers. None have yet been applied to a large vertebrate nervous system. Tract tracing, often described as a "gold standard" in neuroanatomy, suffers from some of the same drawbacks, and it cannot be used in the human brain. At the time of writing, the use of sophisticated diffusion imaging technology offers the most viable road toward mapping the human connectome and understanding its role in behavior and cognition, as well as its dependence on genetic and environmental factors.

Assembling a Large-Scale Network Description

As I have argued from the outset (see chapter 1), one of the most compelling ways to represent connectivity data sets efficiently and compactly is by characterizing them as networks, defined as a set of neural elements and their structural relations, that is, nodes and edges. While formal descriptions of networks in terms of graph theory record mainly topological aspects of the connectivity pattern, the annotation of nodes and edges with spatial (metric) coordinates or measures—for example, node positions or edge lengths—captures important additional information that is invaluable for studies relating network topology to spatial embedding (see chapter 7). Network descriptions are useful regardless of the empirical approach used to map connectome data and regardless of the scale of organization at which connectivity is observed, thus representing a major point of methodological and analytic convergence.

Network descriptions are encountered at all scales. At subcellular scales, neuronal compartments, particularly those forming dendritic arborizations, can be described as graphs (Cuntz et al., 2010; chapter 3; figure 3.1). Dendrites form tree-like structures with numerous linear segments that connect at branch points. Thus, the geometry of dendrites can be formally described by their topology (the relation between branch points and segments, i.e., nodes and edges). Overlaid on this topology are the electrotonic properties of the dendrite, describing how currents flow among its branches and segments. This formulation lends itself to structure–function mappings that can relate morphology to computation within subcellular networks. An interesting possibility is that reconstructions of individual neurons from different cell types will reveal cell-type-specific topologies for these subcellular networks that correspond to the particular signal transformations carried out by these cells.

If such topological classes should exist, they might form important building blocks (akin to motifs) for linking subcellular to circuit-level computation.

Network descriptions are perhaps most conveniently derived at the cellular scale, where nodes and edges naturally correspond to individual cells and their synaptic connections. Asymmetrical chemical synapses correspond to single directed edges, while symmetrical synapses or electrical junctions correspond to bidirectional edges. Once EM and LM approaches to mapping the connectome have identified neurons and their synaptic connections, an important next step will be to reduce the enormous volume of raw data to compact graphs that represent the topology of cellular networks. Some of the first studies in this area have indeed begun to create graphical models (see, e.g., figure 4.4) to report connectivity. Dense reconstructions aim to deliver precise cell-to-cell connection patterns while cellular networks based on statistical descriptions of cell-type-specific connection profiles are inherently probabilistic, with network edges corresponding to likelihoods and densities of connections. As discussed earlier, there is continuing controversy over the value of statistical models of circuits and cell populations, and the outcome of this discussion will likely determine which network description at cellular scales will prevail.

At the large scale, partitioning of the brain into regions defined on the basis of structural criteria such as cytoarchitectonic differences or myelination patterns has a long history. Driven by the influential notion that specific brain functions are localized in specific brain regions, numerous large-scale parcellation schemes for the human brain, particularly cerebral cortex, have been devised.[6] Modern approaches to anatomical parcellation use a wide range of structural criteria. Underlying all these anatomical partitioning approaches is the idea that a region is defined by some structural measure (e.g., cell density, layer structure, receptor or gene expression profiles) that is uniform within regions but distinct from other, particularly neighboring, regions. Once these regions are identified, they are candidates for nodes in large-scale network descriptions. Building on efforts in classical histology, objective and quantitative methods for detecting regional boundaries in cytoarchitecture have been applied to large portions of the human brain with considerable success in refining older partitions derived from largely subjective observations (for a recent study of insular cortex, see Kurth et al., 2010). Additional criteria for regional boundaries come from data on the distribution of important molecules related to neurotransmission such as neurotransmitter receptors (Zilles and Amunts, 2009) and, more recently, from comprehensive gene expression profiles. Building on the first brain-wide gene expression atlas (Ng et al., 2009), Bohland et al. (2010) used clustering techniques to derive a regional partition of the mouse brain based on the regional coherence of gene expression patterns. Regions defined according to their unique gene expression signature showed strong correspondence to anatomical areas defined by classical histology.

Connectome studies employing noninvasive MR strategies require the definition of nodes and edges to derive network descriptions. The smallest spatial unit obtained with noninvasive imaging is the individual volume element (voxel) whose dimensions are entirely defined by parameters of image acquisition. It is important to recall that noninvasive imaging does not allow the observation of individual neurons or circuits and that the voxel partition imposed when images are acquired is arbitrarily placed and does not reflect any underlying neurobiological entities. In addition, the nature of imaging technology often introduces spatial blurring or autocorrelations that are reflected in signal redundancies between neighboring voxels. To create more meaningful partitions requires the aggregation or grouping of voxels into coherent regions according to structural or functional criteria. This is essentially a process of clustering, where the quality of a cluster partition depends on within-cluster coherence and between-cluster separation.

In the context of connectomics, a "good" partition or clustering is one that maximizes information about connectivity. This can be achieved by maximizing specificity and minimizing redundancy in connectivity ascribed to discrete regions. High specificity and low redundancy jointly optimize the uniqueness of each region's connection pattern. Generally, partitions that are too coarse will degrade specificity as regions contain a mixture of connection profiles and information on their origin and destination is lost. Conversely, partitions that are too fine result in high redundancy (as in a voxel-wise partition) since many nodes are simply copies of each other and hence do not contribute unique information. The trade-off between specificity and redundancy can be explored by performing random partitions of the brain into parcels of different size or coarseness. Extremely fine random partitions (down to voxel size) result in larger networks with high redundancy among nodes while coarse random partitions yield smaller networks with low specificity. In general, random partitions are not ideal for connectome studies since they do not respect regional boundaries, thus resulting in an imprecise view of the connection topology and a resultant loss in sensitivity.[7]

At the time of writing, the most commonly used partitioning schemes are based on atlases that use standard coordinates or anatomical landmarks such as characteristic folds or boundaries on the cortical surface. These partitions generally do not correspond to structurally or functionally coherent regions and do not take into account individual data on either connectivity or activation. More recently, a number of innovative techniques for defining coherent brain regions based on data from individual brains have been developed. One set of techniques is based on the observation that different brain regions have different connection profiles, also called "connectional fingerprints" (Passingham et al., 2002) that define their functionality.[8] Data on structural and/or functional connectivity allows the detection of boundaries between regions where connectional profiles change. For example, measurement of the connection profiles over many voxels within a given brain volume (or surface) can be used to compute local gradients of change whose peaks correspond to putative regional boundaries. Another approach is to cluster connection profiles to identify coherent regions, either directly or via their correlation matrix (e.g., Johansen-Berg et al., 2004; figure 5.7, plate 8). Interestingly, it is connectivity itself that leads to an objective definition of the elementary functional units of the human connectome (Knösche and Tittgemeyer, 2011).

Information about brain connectivity used in these approaches can come from either diffusion imaging or resting-state fMRI.[9] Connectivity profiles derived from diffusion imaging have been successfully used to parcellate coherent regions in medial frontal cortex (Johansen-Berg et al., 2004), inferior frontal cortex (Anwander et al., 2007), and cingulate cortex (Beckmann et al., 2009), as well as subcortically for the definition of thalamic nuclei (Johansen-Berg et al., 2005). Gradient-based boundary detection techniques have been applied to resting-state fMRI data (Cohen et al., 2008; figure 5.8). This approach uses algorithms applied in machine vision for image segmentation to detect discontinuities in connection profiles in surface-based cortical maps. In an alternative approach, pattern separation techniques such as independent component analysis (ICA) can be used for detecting voxel clusters with shared covariance structure in resting-state time series data. Complementing approaches based on connectivity are other approaches based on measures of cortical microstructure—for example, patterns of cyto- and myeloarchitecture. Using structural MRI data, Glasser and Van Essen (2011) developed a method for detecting sharp transitions in myelination patterns mapped across the cortical surface. The method could be successfully validated

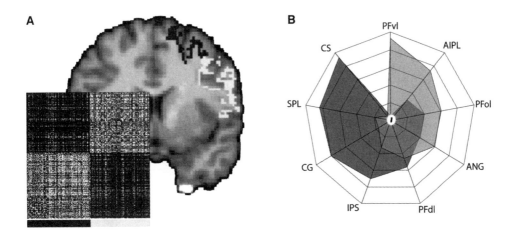

Figure 5.7 (plate 8)
Connectivity-based parcellation of human lateral premotor cortex. (A) The matrix shows
the cross-correlations of the structural connection patterns of voxels in premotor cortex.
The matrix is displayed after clustering to visualize two distinct communities, corresponding to the two sets of voxels displayed in the coronal section. Blue voxels correspond to
putative dorsal premotor cortex (PMd), and red voxels correspond to putative ventral
premotor cortex (PMv). (B) Connectivity fingerprints of PMd (blue) and PMv (red), illustrating the strengths of projections to various regions of parietal and prefrontal cortex.
Projection strength varies from weak (near the center of the plot) to strong (near the
periphery of the plot). PFvl, ventrolateral prefrontal cortex; AIPL, anterior intraparietal
sulcus; PFol, lateral orbital prefrontal cortex; ANG, angular gyrus; PFdl, dorsolateral prefrontal cortex; IPS, medial intraparietal sulcus; CG, cingulate gyrus; SPL, superior parietal
lobule; CS, cingulate sulcus. Reproduced with permission from Johansen-Berg and Rushworth (2009).

on a set of cortical regions whose boundaries were known and in addition
identified numerous new candidates in previously unmapped regions of
cortex.

Several studies have begun to investigate how the joint application of
multiple parcellation criteria can help in identifying coherent brain regions. A combination of resting-state and task-evoked fMRI signals was
used to parcellate lateral parietal cortex (Nelson et al., 2010). The joint
application of gradient detection and network-based modularity partition allowed the identification of anatomically distinct regions. All of
these regions maintained their own characteristic pattern of task activations, thus confirming the distinctiveness of their functional roles. Another study of lateral parietal cortex employed a combination of diffusion
imaging/tractography and resting-state fMRI for mapping both structural and functional connectivity (Mars et al., 2011). After structural
connectivity was used to derive a parcellation into 10 regions, their

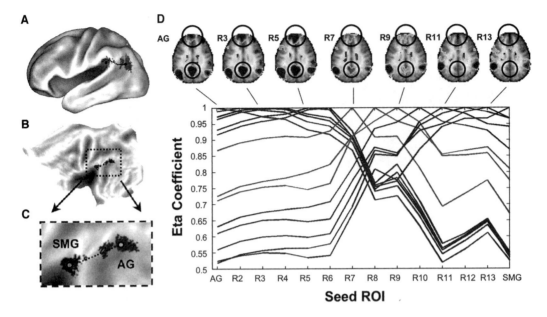

Figure 5.8
Detection of regional boundaries on the basis of resting-state fMRI gradients. Panels A, B, and C show the locations of the supramarginal gyrus (SMG) and the angular gyrus (AG), projected onto an inflated surface of the cerebral cortex (A), and a cortical flat map (B) and (C). The dotted line marks the positions of several seed regions between SMG and AG. (D) Maps at the top represent resting-state functional correlations for several of the seed regions, with circles highlighting parts of the map where connectivity exhibits marked changes across regions. The plot at the bottom represents a measure (eta coefficient) that captures the similarity of connection profiles between each seed pair. For example, the connection profile for seed AG is highly similar to neighboring seeds R2 to R6 and then drops significantly. The combination of multiple similarity patterns defines a gradient where connectivity changes most abruptly, here located in the vicinity of R7 to R9. This location corresponds to a putative regional boundary. ROI, region of interest. Modified (converted to grayscale) and reproduced with permission from Cohen et al. (2008).

functional connectivity profiles were examined and compared. Additionally, a comparison of the architecture of human parietal cortex to that of the macaque monkey was carried out, revealing both similarities and differences.

While a consistent strategy for noninvasive regional parcellation across the human brain has not yet emerged, it appears likely that a combination of multiple structural and functional criteria will be needed to derive robust and maximally informative network descriptions at the large scale. Significant improvements in the definition of network nodes will greatly increase the sensitivity of network analysis across populations of individual participants, thus allowing more sensitive comparisons of network measures with behavioral and genetic variables.

The Two Cultures

The discovery of the human connectome has only just begun. At the time of this writing, no single strategy for mapping the human connectome has crystallized, nor is it likely that a single empirical approach will ever do justice to the multiscale and multifaceted nature of brain connectivity. Instead, it will take the concerted and sustained effort of several different research communities to chart a comprehensive map of the human connectome linking all of its neurons and regions. Different branches of connectomics have begun a process of slow and gradual refinement at all levels, ranging from the reconstruction of spatially highly resolved neurites and synapses in small volumes of neural tissue to the systematic tracing of macroscopic pathways among brain regions. The need for understanding the multiscale nature of the connectome requires growing cooperation and collaboration among scientists who work at different scales in the brain—a merging of the "two cultures" of connectomics aiming at cells and systems.

An important future goal is methodological cross-validation and convergence onto a common description of brain connectivity. In this regard, several opportunities present themselves. EM reconstructions and physiological recordings have already been combined in several recent studies conducted at the microscale (e.g., Bock et al., 2011; Briggman et al., 2011). Validation studies have sought to relate tract tracing and diffusion imaging data in nonhuman primates (e.g., Schmahmann et al., 2007). Other opportunities for cross-scale collaboration exist in the area of segmentation and image reconstruction algorithms which share some of the same logic across all scales—for example, in the definition of neurons in EM sections and in regional parcellation efforts in diffusion imaging. 3D-PLI is a promising new approach leading to data structures that have much in common with diffusion tensor imaging (DTI) and tractography, and both sides stand to gain from sharing computational methods and cross-validating their analyses. Finally, the nascent field of optogenetics applied in animal fMRI (see chapter 6) provides an area of intersection between histology and light microscopy on the one side and noninvasive imaging on the other.

Most of these opportunities for convergence are more easily realized in model organisms since they are invasive and require the manipulation of cells and tissues. This leaves a significant empirical gap for the research enterprise of human connectomics: the establishment of ground truth about circuits and connections in the human brain. For the most part, empirical strategies for mapping the human connectome will have to rely on testing and validation in nonhuman species since the ground truth about neural connections in the human brain will continue to remain largely inaccessible, at least below the level of macroscopic white matter pathways that can be identified in postmortem dissection. This clearly argues for the need to supplement human connectomics with parallel research efforts in model organisms and at all scales. Barring an unforeseen experimental breakthrough, in the near term human connectomics will have to rely on indirect methods to observe connectivity. Such methods require the inference of connectivity models based on observed signal distributions, as for example through the use of tractography in diffusion imaging. It is important to ensure that model inference rests on sound statistical practices and that the validity of inferred connectivity can be tested against new data and predictions. It should be noted that inference comes into play even in microscale connectome strategies such as EM reconstructions because gaps and noise in the data require statistical estimation and error control.

Perhaps the greatest payoff for connectomics will be that it will furnish connectivity models that can explain and predict neural function underlying organismic behavior. Hence, a growing number of empirical studies now focus on "functional connectomics," explicitly combining the recording of neural activity with the conceptual framework of network connectivity. In doing so, the complex functioning of the connectome in circuits and systems is beginning to be revealed. We now turn to the new challenges that are encountered as we consider the connectome in motion.

6 The Connectome in Motion

Like genes, structural connections alone are powerless. The causal efficacy of genes and connections depends on their functional expression as part of complex biological networks. Genomic sequences come to life through transcriptional and protein networks which are essential for organizing cellular metabolism and for creating differentiated cells, tissues, and organs. Similarly, the connectome must be expressed in dynamic neural activity to be effective in behavior and cognition. How this is accomplished is far from trivial. Given the nature of networked systems, each of the elements and connections of the brain contributes to multiple functional domains and outcomes. Establishing how the structure of brain networks translates into behavior is therefore a particularly challenging research goal for human connectomics. This chapter summarizes our current knowledge about how the connectome shapes the dynamics of neural activity, the changing pattern of functional relations between neural elements unfolding on multiple time scales.

The connectome is both the source and the target of brain dynamics. Its topology enables specific neural interactions and is thus a major factor in generating patterns of functional connectivity (figure 6.1). At the same time, connectome topology is subject to neuroplasticity inscribing lasting traces of past events and experience (see chapter 3). This mutual interaction of topology and dynamics introduces the element of time. Plasticity renders the topological structure of the connectome time dependent, and neural activity gives rise to a rich set of time-varying patterns which can be described as a set of functional networks. These functional networks depend not only on the connectome's structural linkages but on powerful modulation by changes in the internal state of the organism and by the momentary demands of the external environment. Thus, the structure of the connectome turns into dynamic patterns

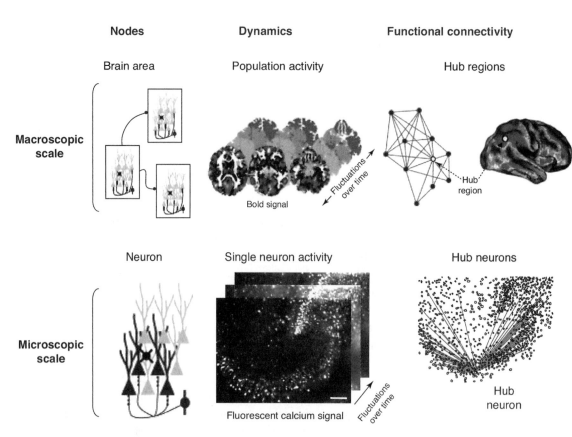

Nodes   **Dynamics**   **Functional connectivity**

Brain area   Population activity   Hub regions

Macroscopic scale

Bold signal

Hub region

Neuron   Single neuron activity   Hub neurons

Microscopic scale

Fluorescent calcium signal

Fluctuations over time

Hub neuron

Figure 6.1
Functional connectivity at different levels of organization. At the top, networks of brain regions give rise to population dynamics that can be observed with functional magnetic resonance imaging (Bold signal; blood oxygenation level dependent signal). At the bottom, networks of individual neurons give rise to activity patterns that can be observed with optical imaging or neurophysiological methods. In both cases, the resulting neural time series can be processed as functional connectivity which allows the detection of conspicuous highly connected hub regions or hub neurons. Modified (converted to grayscale) and reproduced with permission from Feldt et al. (2011).

that are essential for the temporal continuity of sensorimotor activity and cognitive processes.

The dynamic nature of the connectome has a close parallel in systems biology. Cellular processes depend on networks of dynamic interactions between molecular components, including RNA transcripts, proteins, and metabolites. These dynamic networks represent the cell's "functional connectivity," and their state dependence and time dependence is an emerging research focus (Przytycka et al., 2010).[1] It is through these dynamic patterns that genetic information is "read out" (a form of decoding) and gives rise to biological forms and functions. The nature of these dynamic networks makes it difficult, if not impossible, to relate individual genetic elements to specific phenotypic traits of organisms. For connectomics, a principal challenge for the future is to understand how information encoded in neural wiring becomes expressed in cognition and behavior, and it seems likely that the challenge will be at least as difficult as the one currently faced in genomics. Nevertheless, a beginning is made as our increasing knowledge about the human connectome starts to link up with the investigation of functional brain states and their dynamic networks.

The Structural Basis of Functional Connectivity

Brain recordings yield time series of neural activity that can be captured by a wide range of signals from neural spike trains to field potentials and hemodynamic responses. Neural activations and their time courses often display highly characteristic statistical patterns, encoding specific information in relation to external inputs, varying with the internal state of the organism, and reflecting past experience and future expectations. These highly specific response properties are in part due to specific patterns in the brain's structural connectivity, its connectome. Structural connections channel the signal flow between network elements and thus contribute to observed neural activations and interactions.

The strength and pattern of neuronal interactions can be estimated from observed brain dynamics with a broad range of measures and techniques. Recordings of neural time series are usually obtained from multiple neural elements represented by sets of individual neurons or neural populations, field potential electrodes, electromagnetic sensors, or neuroimaging voxels. Numerous analysis methods are available for estimating statistical dependencies or dynamic interactions from time series data recorded from multiple neural elements. Once these dependencies have been computed they can be converted into a connectivity matrix representing a functional brain network (see chapter 1).[2] For most measures, functional connections can vary in magnitude on a continuous scale, and if they are expressed as linear cross-correlations they can have positive or negative sign. It is important to note that unlike structural connectivity, which refers to an objectively verifiable pattern of anatomical links, functional networks are statistical constructs that exhibit considerable variability on short time scales, either spontaneously (see figure 2.3) or in response to varying conditions of input and task (e.g., Moussa et al., 2011). Thus, the number of possible configurations of functional connections far exceeds the number of underlying structural connections. This once again underscores the important distinction between the connectome itself and its dynamics. Functional connections reflect network dynamics unfolding within or emerging from the connectome's structural substrate.

Statistical dependencies can exist regardless of whether two neural elements are anatomically linked or not[3] and thus do not reflect structural connectivity in any simple way. While statistical dependencies are often easily computed from time series data, they do not allow solid inferences about causal interactions. In contrast, such interactions may be revealed by effective connectivity, generally defined as a set of causal relations between neural elements or, more specifically, as a network representing a generative model underlying observed data (see chapter 1; table 1.1). This definition differs considerably from the much broader, fundamentally acausal and model-free nature of functional connectivity. Yet, even if one considers effective connectivity, the causal relations it describes are continually modulated by endogenous transitions in internal state as well as exogenous perturbations of inputs and task set. Hence, effective connectivity, like functional connectivity, emerges from the human connectome as a large repertoire of variable relationships among neural elements. Effective connectivity has a long history in systems neuroscience, beginning with the first applications of statistical techniques designed to extract directed neural interactions in neurophysiology and human imaging studies (e.g., Aertsen et al., 1989; McIntosh et al., 1994). Since then, research on effective connectivity has proceeded along several paths, including lag-based measures such as Granger causality (now often classified as a measure of functional connectivity) as well as Bayesian model selection approaches. For now, I will focus the discussion on simple measures of functional connectivity described by correlations of neural events recorded over time.

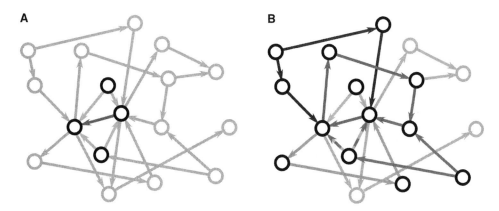

Figure 6.2 (plate 9)
Sources of correlations in neural activity. Circles represent neural elements and arrows represent directed synaptic connections. We consider the pair of neurons indicated by red circles. (A) Correlations between these two neurons can be due to a direct synaptic connection (dark blue arrow), or common input from directly connected elements (light blue arrows). (B) In addition, network-wide effects can play a role, including indirect paths of synaptic connections (orange, yellow) and indirect common input (light and dark green). Nodes and connections shaded in gray cannot exert any influence on the two red circles. The nature of network-wide effects on local correlations is the same at the microscale and at the macroscale. Reproduced from Pernice et al. (2011).

The nature of the relationship between observed neural correlations and the underlying structural network has become a topic of investigation in both empirical and computational studies. The revival of circuit anatomy has stimulated a number of studies attempting to relate spike patterns to the topological layout of synaptic connections. In a network setting, the relative timing of spikes and the resulting cross-correlations depend on multiple types of effects, including direct and indirect interactions, and common input (figure 6.2, plate 9). Modeling studies have examined how different connection topologies can induce pairwise correlations among spiking neurons (Pernice et al., 2011). In networks with random topology that is either uniform or distance dependent, average pairwise correlations were found to be low and highly variable. Mutual connections between highly connected hub neurons increased average correlations, and similar increases were seen in topologies where neurons were organized into highly connected local patches. Overall, not only did different architectures exhibit different levels of pairwise correlations but different local motifs were found to make different contributions to the observed distribution of dynamic couplings.

Neural recordings of cells in sensory cortices have generally reported a preponderance of weak average correlations, even among neurons that exhibit similar stimulus preferences (Ecker et al., 2010; Renart et al., 2010), implying active decorrelation through recurrent and inhibitory mechanisms. Closer analysis of correlations across different spatial scales in macaque visual cortex revealed that correlation patterns are scale-dependent (Ohiorhenuan et al., 2010). At fine scales of a few hundred micrometers, visual stimuli induced rapid reconfigurations of correlations while neurons separated by longer distances remained only weakly correlated. These local effects are presumed to result from nonrandom features of synaptic connectivity, including the observed abundance of specific network motifs (Song et al., 2005). Such network motifs can generate specific patterns of connectivity that drive functional specificity. An analysis of synaptic connections between mouse visual cortical neurons demonstrated higher numbers of structural connections between neurons with similar response preferences, as well as a greater incidence of bidirectional connections than expected by chance (Ko et al., 2011), consistent with correlation patterns observed in physiological recordings (Ch'ng and Reid, 2010). Other empirical studies have attempted to directly relate reconstructed neural circuits to specific functional properties of neurons (see chapter 4; Briggman et al., 2011; Bock et al., 2011). Consistently, specific patterns of structural connections were associated with specific physiological response properties or interactions among neurons. These studies represent initial forays into "functional connectomics," an area of research that attempts to establish links between patterns of structural connectivity and the statistics of neural responses through correlated observations of circuit structure and function.

A very similar approach, albeit at a different scale, has documented significant relationships between structural and functional connectivity in whole-brain MRI (Honey et al., 2010). Hemodynamic signal fluctuations recorded during the brain's resting-state are readily processed into networks of cross-correlations between nodes, either individual voxels or parcellated regions (Bullmore and Sporns, 2009). Aggregated over the whole brain, this analysis yields resting-state functional connectivity matrices that describe statistical dependencies averaged over relatively long sampling epochs (often on the order of 6–10 minutes). An abundance of empirical studies has shown that these longtime averages disclose the architecture of human neurocognitive networks in remarkable detail (see the next section). It appears that the stability and consistency of these functional patterns can partly be traced to underlying patterns of structural connectivity. A landmark study conducted in macaque monkey cerebral cortex first provided compelling evidence for significant overlap between neuroanatomical connections and correlations in fMRI signals (Vincent et al., 2007; figure 6.3, plate 10). In humans, Hagmann et al. (2008) compared whole-brain structural networks derived from diffusion MRI and functional networks acquired during the resting state. Key to the comparison was that both networks were mapped onto the same brain parcellation and compared within the same set of individual participants. A more detailed analysis (Honey et al., 2009; figure 6.4) demonstrated that the presence and strength of a structural connection significantly predicted the strength of a functional connection across all node pairs. Furthermore, a computational model of neural populations with structural couplings derived from diffusion MRI could substantially reproduce the empirically observed fMRI functional connectivity (see chapter 8). Thus, it appears it is possible, up to a degree, to predict resting-state functional networks from structural networks. However, the reverse inference of structural couplings from functional connections turned out to be impractical due to the high base rate of false positives when thresholding to retain strong functional links. The density of strong functional connections is far greater than the density of structural connections, reflecting the propensity of statistical correlations to span nodes that are structurally only indirectly connected. Nevertheless, despite the impossibility of reverse inference, a plausible hypothesis suggests that all functional connections are ultimately caused by the structural links comprising the connectome, through a combination of direct and indirect network effects.

In rare cases, experimental manipulations of the human connectome can be directly linked to concomitant alterations in functional connectivity. Callosotomy is a surgical procedure performed in some cases to treat intractable epilepsy. It involves the complete sectioning of the corpus callosum and thus interrupts most direct structural connections between the two cortical hemispheres.[4] The role of callosal connections in generating interhemispheric functional connectivity was directly demonstrated by performing mapping of resting-state functional connectivity before and after the procedure was performed in a single 6-year-old patient (Johnston et al., 2008; figure 6.5, plate 11). Before callosotomy, strong interhemispheric functional connectivity linked corresponding regions in frontal and parietal cortex. Immediately after surgery, these functional connections had disappeared while intrahemispheric functional

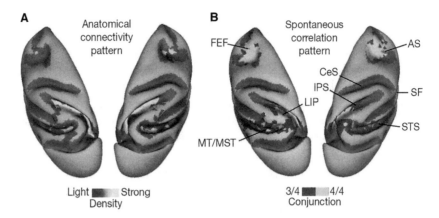

Figure 6.3 (plate 10)
Anatomical and functional connectivity in macaque parietal and frontal cortex. Anatomical connectivity was determined from tracer injections, and functional connectivity is represented as blood oxygen level dependent (BOLD) cross-correlations, recorded during spontaneous brain activity under anesthesia. Both panels show data displayed on the top surface of the two macaque cerebral hemispheres. (A) A map of retrogradely labeled brain regions after injection into the lateral intraparietal area (LIP). (B) A map of voxels exhibiting BOLD correlations among at least three out of four regions of the monkey oculomotor system (FEF, frontal eye fields; LIP; MT, middle temporal area; MST, middle superior temporal area). AS, arcuate sulcus; CeS, central sulcus; IPS, intraparietal sulcus; SF, sylvian fissure; STS, superior temporal sulcus. Adapted and reproduced with permission from Vincent et al. (2007).

connections were largely unperturbed.[5] This rare case of direct manipulation of a major pathway in the human connectome directly demonstrates the important role of structural connections in generating functional connectivity. The effect of callosotomy on interhemispheric functional connectivity can be reproduced in a computational model (see figure 6.5; chapter 8).

Numerous other studies have documented the relation between structural and functional connectivity in human brain recordings (e.g., Skudlarski et al., 2008; Greicius et al., 2009; van den Heuvel et al., 2009a). Not only are structure–function relations of interest in the healthy brain, they can be of particular value in conditions where functional disruptions can be traced to a structural cause. A large number of studies of patient populations have shown disturbed functional connectivity, and such disturbances are often attributed to "miswiring," a physical or structural alteration of the connectome. Systematic and correlated structure–function studies in brain disorders are promising but have yet to be carried out in a systematic way. Another important target of investigation

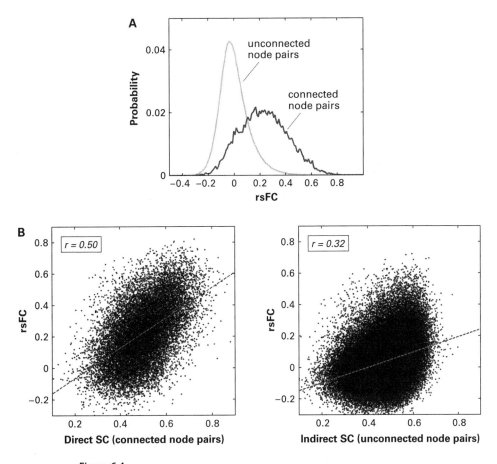

Figure 6.4
Relation of structural to functional connectivity. The data plotted here are comparing structural connectivity (SC) and resting-state functional connectivity (rsFC) among 998 regions of interest (nodes) randomly partitioning the cerebral cortex (Hagmann et al., 2008) (A) Histograms of the strength of rsFC between pairs of regions that are linked by a structural connection ("connected node pairs") and pairs of regions for which direct SC is absent ("unconnected node pairs"). Since structural connections are sparse, there are far more unconnected than connected node pairs. Note that the two distributions overlap, with numerous instances of strong rsFC between unconnected node pairs. (B) Scatter plots of direct SC and indirect SC (computed as the sum of the product of edge weights along all paths of length 2), and rsFC. Both relationships are significant at $p < 0.001$ and indicate that direct as well as indirect SC is partially predictive of rsFC. Data replotted from Hagmann et al. (2008).

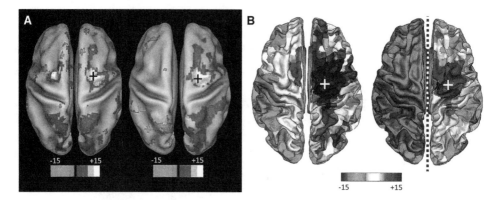

Figure 6.5 (plate 11)

Functional connectivity before and after callosotomy. Both sets of images show a z-score correlation map of resting-state functional magnetic resonance imaging seeded in the vicinity of the frontal eye fields located in the right cortical hemisphere (marked "+"). (A) Empirical recordings from a human patient before (left) and after (right) transection of the corpus callosum. Preoperatively, positive functional connectivity extends across the frontal and parietal cortex in both hemispheres. Postoperatively, functional connectivity is restricted to the right hemisphere, and interhemispheric functional connectivity is largely absent. Figure modified and reproduced with permission from Johnston et al. (2008). (B) Simulated functional connectivity from a computational model of the human brain (Honey et al., 2009) with an intact (left) and cut (right) corpus callosum. Note the lack of functional connectivity between hemispheres.

is brain development. Two independent studies have examined the normal development of the structure–function relationship in the human cerebral cortex (Hagmann et al., 2010b; Supekar et al., 2010). Both studies found evidence for a progressive strengthening of structural pathways, particularly those linking remote brain regions, and concomitant changes in functional interactions. In addition, Hagmann et al. (2010b) reported that the degree to which structural connections predicted functional connections strengthened over developmental time. This pattern may reflect the protracted time course for maturation of pathways or greater variability of signal fluctuations at early developmental stages.

Several points deserve to be emphasized (and some will be taken up in more detail in the next two chapters). First, these results confirm the important predictive power of structural connections for physiological responses, and the value of an accurate structural model for "forward computation" of neural activity patterns. This is the main rationale for the construction of computational models that are akin to a "virtual brain." Second, the inverse problem of inferring a structural network from dynamic time series recordings generally cannot be solved, at least not with simple "model-free" approaches like thresholding.[6] Functional connectivity alone is insufficient as it is generally derived from brain signal fluctuations without reference to a generative model, and its origin is thus structurally and causally unspecified. Instead, model-based approaches stand a much better chance at providing a principled solution to the problem. A strategy based on Bayesian model selection applied to families of generative models that are evaluated in the context of task-evoked or resting brain activity has been successfully deployed in brain network discovery (Friston et al., 2011). We will explore the dual roles of forward modeling and model inference further in chapter 8.

An entirely different way to probe the structure–function relationship is offered by approaches that introduce a local perturbation or an external stimulus and observe its effects across brain regions, presumably mediated by structural pathways. These perturbational approaches permit more direct inferences of causal relations between network elements, particularly if results from multiple perturbations are combined into a coherent network model. In humans, perturbations are most often performed by applying sensory stimulation or imposing task conditions. More invasive perturbations include the use of transcranial magnetic stimulation (TMS). TMS can selectively disrupt sensory and cognitive processing, and its effects on neural activity can be mapped with simultaneous EEG recordings. Using this approach, it has been shown that identical TMS perturbations can have different neural effects depending on the global state of the brain—for example, when applied in different stages of waking, sleep, and anesthesia (Massimini et al., 2005; Ferrarelli et al., 2010). Perturbations travel more widely and involve a larger set of brain regions remote to the site of stimulation during waking whereas their effects remain much more localized during sleep and anesthesia.

Another opportunity for targeted perturbations and causal network mapping is provided by direct stimulation of specific cell populations. In animal models, the use of optogenetic techniques (Boyden et al., 2005) renders specific cell populations responsive to light through the targeted introduction of a microbial light-sensitive membrane protein. Application of light stimuli allows the temporally precise activation (or deactivation) of specific brain regions. Extending the approach to fMRI in the rat brain, Lee et al. (2010) recorded hemodynamic signals both locally within a stimulated region and in other regions known to be anatomically linked. In an extension of the technique to mouse brain, targeted stimulation of cortical pyramidal cells has been shown to evoke interregional functional connectivity in BOLD signals (Desai et al., 2011). These experiments lend additional support to the notion that BOLD functional connectivity is caused by neural signal flow in the structural circuits of the connectome. Opto-fMRI may thus open the door to causal mapping and activation of specific circuits in live animals (Lee, 2011) and may perhaps even provide a new way to deliver therapeutic deep-brain stimulation in humans.

The neural elements and connections comprising the complex network of the human brain contribute to its operation in ways that transcend simple one-to-one structure–function relations. Despite this complexity, evidence from cellular and systems-level studies suggests that structural connectivity can indeed predict statistical interactions between neurons and brain regions as well as their specific physiological and functional properties. In the human brain, the functional networks derived from spontaneous fluctuations of the BOLD signal during rest have received significant attention, for they have proven to be extraordinarily informative about brain organization.

Functional Modules and Neurocognitive Networks

Resting-state fMRI generally involves the collection of BOLD time series over a period of several minutes while the person is quietly awake and cognitively at rest. Resting-state functional connectivity is then derived from statistical dependencies between the time series, most commonly expressed as their cross-correlation. Despite the unconstrained nature of "quiet rest," functional connectivity exhibits characteristic patterns of interactions that are consistent within and across individual participants (Fox and Raichle, 2007; van den Heuvel and Hulshoff Pol, 2010; Raichle, 2011). These patterns have proven extremely useful in the analysis of brain organization and connectivity in healthy adults, as well as in developing and diseased brains.[7] The neuronal basis for low-frequency spontaneous fluctuations of the BOLD response observed in the resting state remains a matter of continued investigation. Recent work has established a strong link between BOLD fluctuations and oscillations in power and synchrony of neural activity (Nir et al., 2008; Shmuel and Leopold, 2008; Schölvinck et al., 2010), but the origin of these fluctuations and the mechanisms by which they are translated into hemodynamic signals are yet to be fully uncovered.

The utility of resting-state fMRI for human connectomics derives from its consistency across individual participants (Damoiseaux et al., 2006), test–retest reliability (van Dijk et al., 2010), relative stability over time

(Shehzad et al., 2009) and across changes in brain state including awareness (Boly et al., 2008), its dependable developmental time course (Fair et al., 2009), heritability (Glahn et al., 2010), and characteristic alterations in various states of brain disease (Zhang and Raichle, 2010; Bassett and Bullmore, 2009). Network and cluster analysis of resting-state functional connectivity has revealed a number of "resting-state networks" (RSNs) consisting of spatially distributed and interconnected brain regions that form core functional modules. Most prominent among these is a set of brain regions including the precuneus/posterior cingulate cortex, lateral parietal cortex, and medial frontal cortex whose neuronal and metabolic activity is elevated at rest (Raichle et al., 2001), and that are mutually interconnected to form the "default mode network" (Greicius et al., 2003; Buckner et al., 2008). Other networks are involved in mediating attention, cognitive control, salience, and motor and sensory processing (Damoiseaux et al., 2006; De Luca et al., 2006). When one is mapping functional connections within and between RSNs, they appear as distinct modules whose elements are strongly linked within modules and are less strongly linked between modules (Raichle, 2011; figure 6.6, plate 12).

Various clustering, modularity, or segmentation approaches applied to resting-state fMRI are beginning to converge on a consistent set of resting-state networks that comprise the building blocks of spontaneous and task-evoked brain dynamics. Two of the leading segmentation techniques are network-based partitioning into functional modules and the detection of temporally independent components. The spatial resolution of both approaches depends in part on parameters governing data acquisition and postprocessing like run length, voxel dimensions, elimination of physiological noise and movement artifacts. Hence there is no final agreement yet across methods and experimental procedures on the inventory of large-scale human functional networks. Three recent studies that have attempted to map these networks across the human brain have reported largely consistent findings. Doucet et al. (2011) identified 23 RSNs in a sample of 180 participants. These RSNs were arranged hierarchically, with two very extensive anticorrelated systems associated with "intrinsic" versus "extrinsic" processing at the top of the hierarchy (figure 6.7, plate 13). Yeo et al. (2011) partitioned the cerebral cortex into a smaller number of RSNs using a clustering algorithm, deriving a coarse partition into 7 networks and a finer partition into 17 networks from a total of 1,000 individual data sets. Power et al. (2011) used modularity detection to identify coherent networks called subgraphs in resting-state

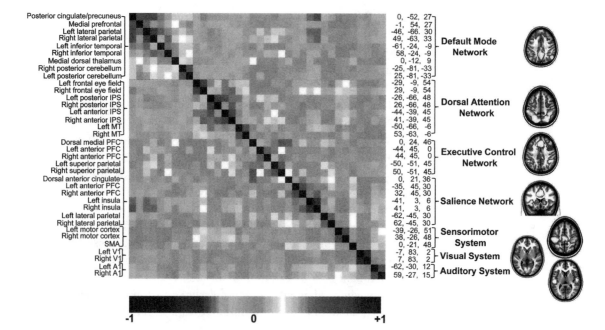

Figure 6.6 (plate 12)

Seven resting-state brain networks and their interconnections. The seven networks are displayed at the right of the diagram, with their central regions of interest listed at the left. The matrix shows BOLD signal cross-correlations obtained from a single 30-minute period of resting brain activity recorded from a healthy adult male participant. Note the distinctive block structure of the correlation matrix, indicative of mostly strong and positive correlations within each network. Note also that some degree of correlation persists between networks. A movie showing windowed cross-correlation and illustrating the waxing and waning of correlations within and between networks can be found at ftp://imaging.wustl.edu/pub/raichlab/restless_brain. IPS, inferior parietal sulcus; MT, middle temporal area; PFC, prefrontal cortex; SMA, supplementary motor area; V1, visual area 1; A1, auditory area 1. Reproduced with permission from Raichle (2011).

fMRI data and in many cases established correspondence between these RSNs and functional subsystems previously identified on the basis of task activations. Taken together, the results from these studies suggest that most networks identified in resting brain activity can be associated with specific cognitive or behavioral domains. While it is certainly tempting to stress the functional specialization of these networks, it is also important to note that they do not operate in isolation from one another. Partitioned modules or networks are found to share interconnecting nodes and edges that are of critical importance for the global functional coherence of the cortical system. These hub nodes or edges are the articulation points of the cortical architecture.

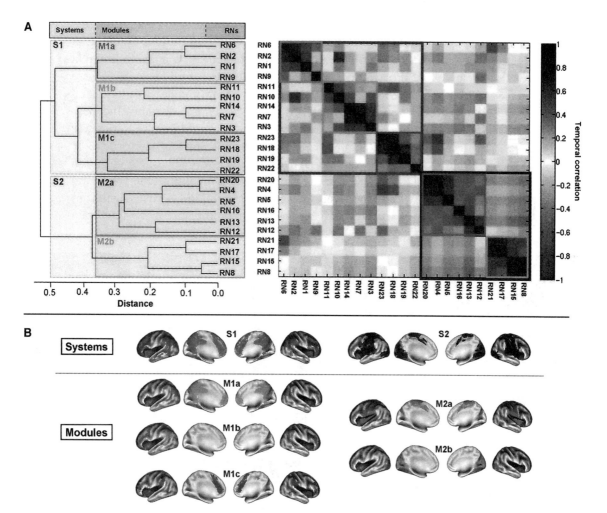

Figure 6.7 (plate 13)
Hierarchical clustering of resting-state networks. A total of 22 resting networks (RNs) were identified by independent components analysis carried out on 8-minute resting-state functional magnetic resonance imaging blood oxygen level dependent time series acquired from a total of 180 participants (Doucet et al., 2011). (A) The dendrogram at the left was constructed on the basis of temporal correlations of resting-state networks, averaged over all participants. The first levels of the dendrogram revealed two global systems (S1, S2) and five modules (M1a, M1b, M1c for S1; M2a, M2b for S2). The averaged temporal correlations are displayed at the right. (B) Spatial maps of systems and modules (cf. figure 6.6 and 6.8). Module M1a comprises a number of default mode regions, including the posterior cingulate/precuneus and parts of medial frontal and lateral parietal cortex. Module M2b consists mostly of occipital (visual) regions. Modified and reproduced with permission from Doucet et al. (2011).

Importantly, the functional architecture disclosed by signal fluctuations at rest is consistent with coactivation patterns observed under task demands (Smith et al., 2009). Thousands of activation maps collected in a large repository of task-based imaging studies (Laird et al., 2005) were used to derive covariance patterns that identify coherently activated brain regions in the context of specific behavioral domains. Independently, the covariance structure of resting-state fMRI time series was used to identify coherent subnetworks as independent components in brain dynamics. A common set of networks was identified, and each network was found to be associated with a unique set of behavioral domains (figure 6.8; see also chapter 8 and figure 8.6). The significant similarity between the two sets of networks implies that resting brain

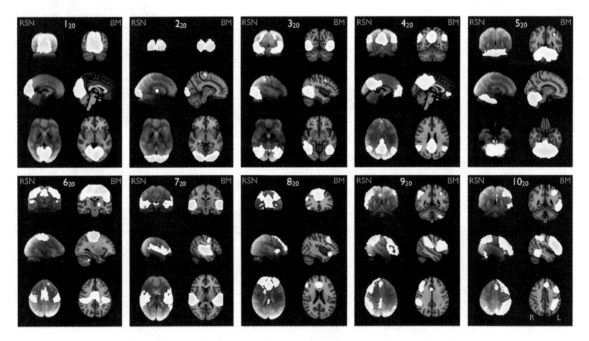

Figure 6.8
Networks extracted from resting-state and task-evoked activation data. Each of the 10 panels shows two matched independent components (based on a 20-component independent components analysis [ICA], displayed in three informative orthogonal slices each, oriented along the coronal, sagittal, and horizontal planes). The components were extracted from resting-state fMRI data (RSN) and the BrainMap database of neuroimaging activation studies (BM). ICA spatial maps were thresholded at z = 3 and are shown here as bright areas overlaid on standard brain images. Their association with different domains of cognition and behavior is shown in figure 8.6. Modified (converted to grayscale) and reproduced with permission from Smith et al. (2009).

dynamics involves a succession or "rehearsal" of a repertoire of task-related functional networks. This consistency in functional network architecture across task and rest conditions strongly points to a shared structural basis in the topology of the large-scale connectome. A plausible hypothesis suggests that the composition and covariance structure of large-scale functional networks is the product of dynamic processes unfolding on a specific structural connection pattern.

Resting-state functional connectivity as measured with fMRI exhibits experience-dependent changes over time, possibly the result of synaptic plasticity. Intense practice of a visual perceptual learning task was found to induce changes in the pattern of resting-state BOLD signal fluctuations in specific and task-related functional networks (Lewis et al., 2009). These results are consistent with other studies reporting modulation of resting-state BOLD functional connectivity by recent experience (Stevens et al., 2010; Grigg and Grady, 2010). The relation to plasticity may illuminate possible functional roles of spontaneous neural activity in preserving and continually rehearsing traces of sensory and motor experience. The history of regional coactivation during behavior results in the differential modification of structural links that, in turn, become engaged during spontaneous neural activity (Power et al., 2011). Resting-state correlations may thus partly reflect accumulated experience traces that have become inscribed in the structure of the connectome. At rest, the connectome enables spontaneous neural activity that actively rehearses past mental states, a powerful process of reactivation and consolidation that is largely hidden from consciousness.

Thus, resting-state functional connectivity can be regarded as a robust neural trait reflecting both genetic and experiential modifications of the connectome. While the global pattern is largely held in common across participants, important individual differences in connectivity, driven by heritable variation and environmental experience, jointly underpin individual differences in behavior. Given their consistency, functional networks recorded in the resting state are uniquely relevant for human connectomics as they allow rapid, reproducible, and noninvasive assessment of brain architecture, potentially across very large numbers of human participants. Building on this premise, Biswal et al. (2010) have suggested that resting-state fMRI may present a general paradigm for mapping individual brain architecture, referred to as the "functional connectome." In an unprecedented effort involving the sharing and public posting of over a thousand neuroimaging data sets from across 35 globally distributed MRI centers, Biswal and colleagues demonstrated both the universality and the individual variability of resting-state functional networks. Pooled data from the 1000 Functional Connectomes Project has since been mined and analyzed in numerous other studies directed at finding patterns of variation and developing new analysis tools. The creation of an open-access data repository of this magnitude and geographic range is significant for other reasons as well (see chapter 8). It complements the prevailing research model of collecting data from relatively small-scale investigations and marks the arrival of large-scale discovery science in human neuroimaging. Here, emphasis is placed on collecting and disseminating large data sets with the goal of generating new hypotheses and integrating data across research domains, including imaging, behavior, and genetics. The impending availability of thousands and perhaps tens of thousands of functional connectivity data sets will allow the exploration of brain–behavior relationships and of genetic influences on brain architecture at an unprecedented scale.

Particularly promising is the integration of structural and functional connectome data with data that relate to tissue metabolism and gene expression. Functional neuroimaging depends on the transduction of neural activity into a hemodynamic signal and is thus closely associated with mechanisms of neurovascular coupling, local tissue metabolism, and energy consumption. The high energy demands of the brain[8] place tight constraints on the availability and utilization of energy in response to neural activity. Various considerations of cellular processes involving the consumption of glucose, oxygen, and ATP lead to the conclusion that much of the brain's metabolic energy is devoted to non-task-dependent or intrinsic neural activity (Raichle and Mintun, 2006). Of particular interest in the current context are regional variations in some metabolic processes such as glycolysis as measured by positron emission tomography (PET; Vaishnavi et al., 2010; figure 6.9, plate 14). Aerobic glycolysis refers to the partial breakdown of glucose in the presence of oxygen, but without engaging a chain of reactions called oxidative phosphorylation whose ultimate products are carbon dioxide and water. It is commonly found in cancer cells as well as in highly active brain tissue where the level of glycolysis exhibits regional fluctuations accompanying both task-evoked and resting brain activity. Interestingly, high levels of aerobic glycolysis are associated with specific brain networks, particularly those involved in the default mode and in cognitive control (Vaishnavi et al., 2010). Regional levels of anaerobic glycolysis are also found to be correlated with regional centrality in the brain's structural networks

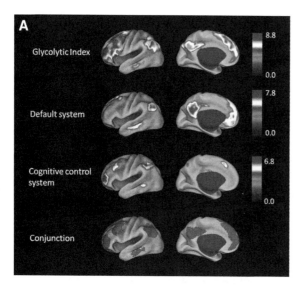
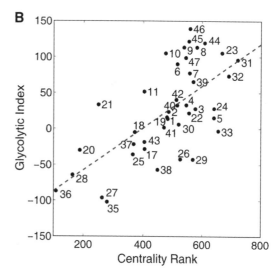

Figure 6.9 (plate 14)
Relation between brain metabolism and network architecture. (A) Panels show (top to bottom) regional distribution of aerobic glycolysis measured by the glycolytic index (Vaishnavi et al., 2010), the default mode system and the cognitive control system measured by resting-state functional magnetic resonance imaging mapping, and a conjunction of the top panel with the union of the two middle panels illustrating their overlap. Image reproduced with permission from Vaishnavi et al. (2010). (B) A scatter plot of the centrality rank, estimated from the betweenness centrality of the connectomes of five participants reported in Hagmann et al. (2008), and the glycolytic index as reported in Vaishnavi et al. (2010), for 41 Brodmann areas of cerebral cortex. Higher centrality rank indicates that the region participates in a larger number of short communication paths in the structural network. High centrality is a key criterion for a structural hub. The correlation is highly significant, with r = 0.66 (p < 10^{-5}).

(Hagmann et al., 2008; see figure 6.9).[9] Given that high centrality is a central feature of hub regions, the association suggests the hypothesis that hubs differ in their energy metabolism with respect to other less central regions of the brain. Thus, structural connectivity patterns may not only impact neural processing but also drive metabolic cost and demand.[10] It is to be expected that the availability of large imaging data sets through efforts like the 1000 Functional Connectomes and the Human Connectome Project will be instrumental in bringing about a new level of integration across multiple structural and functional data domains defining the human brain in terms of connectivity, metabolism, energy utilization, and gene expression.

As this brief survey shows, the future goals of functional connectomics are highly complementary to parallel efforts to map the structural connections of the human brain. Functional connectomics captures networks of dynamic interactions in order to characterize invariant and characteristic features of brain organization. However, it is important to remember that when estimated from signals acquired over relatively long observation periods (several minutes in the case of resting-state fMRI), the strengths of functional connections only provide information about average levels of interactions. Connections (edges) that appear weak on a time scale of minutes may show intermittent periods of strong dynamic linkage or even switch between positive and negative coupling. Such "edge dynamics" are revealed only when functional connectivity is estimated from brief time windows. Average estimates of dynamic couplings on a time scale of minutes provide only limited information about how these couplings relate to cognitive processes, commonly thought to occur on time scales of tens and hundreds of milliseconds. While observing functional connectivity at fast time scales presents many technical and analytical challenges, it is an essential step toward characterizing the connectional substrate of cognition.

Variable Neural Dynamics and the Functional Repertoire

As neuronal and regional activations fluctuate on fast time scales, networks defined by their covariance or causal dependency undergo equally fast temporal modulations. These fast modulations and reconfigurations of functional networks are of central importance for understanding information flow and computation in the brain. Computation, when viewed from the network perspective, is the dynamic generation and integration of information in a connected system resulting in coordinated neural population activity. These coordinated states are associated with functional networks and their dynamic changes through time. Changing network topology will be reflected in fluctuations of local and global network measures that assess the balance between local (segregated) and global (integrated) processing as well as the contributions of regions and pathways to network-wide dynamics. Since neural computation is so closely tied to network dynamics, it is important to discover the driving force behind variability in brain functional networks.

Before we explore this question more fully, we first need to make a crucial distinction between fluctuations that arise from stochastic or random processes and those that arise from nonlinear dynamics. Stochasticity generates noise, defined as random and undesirable disturbances of signals. Noise can have many origins, from thermal noise in ion movements, to cellular variations in number or arrangement of molecular components, stochastic signal transmission at synapses, activation of sensory receptors or recruitment of motor circuits. Such stochastic noise is often viewed as an unwanted corruption of true signal components. But noise driven by stochastic processes at microscales can contribute to variability in macroscopic neural and behavioral responses. Additionally, large-scale dynamic variability can arise even in an entirely deterministic system if the system is sensitive to small differences in initial conditions, a hallmark of chaos. Jointly, stochastic fluctuations and dynamic variability may well be regarded as "signal," in the sense that they become manifest in macroscopic system behavior and contribute to the system's functional capability (Deco and Corbetta, 2011).

Much of the recent work in functional brain networks has focused on identifying consistent and stable dynamic patterns—for example, in the course of spontaneous resting-state activity. More recently, the extent and possible functional role of variability in brain dynamics has received renewed attention. This recent work is building on a long history of research on variable brain dynamics, particularly in electrophysiology. Despite this rich body of work, how variable dynamics arises from brain connectivity has remained elusive. On fast time scales, several recent reports have documented nonstationary dynamics of functional connectivity in EEG and MEG recordings. Unlike stationary processes whose statistical parameters remain stable across time, nonstationary dynamics exhibits significant fluctuations in the probability distributions of system states. Nonstationarity can be tracked by recording changes in the dynamic association between nodes, essentially creating edge time series data for statistical measures of their dependence or causal interactions. These edge time series, when aggregated among a set of nodes, define time-varying networks of functional interactions.

Analyzing the spatial distribution of electric potentials generated by human brain activity, Dietrich Lehmann developed the concept of "EEG microstates," brief episodes of stability lasting on the order of 100 milliseconds (Lehmann et al., 1987; Lehmann, 1990). These stable distributions of electric potentials are interspersed with rapid transitions, rendering the system overall quasi- or metastable. EEG microstates can be classified into a small set of patterns, and they unfold across time in specific sequences that are thought to reflect the momentary fluctuations of mental processing.[11] Recent work has established a link between spontaneously occurring EEG microstates and resting-state brain dynamics as recorded by fMRI. In simultaneous EEG/fMRI recordings, specific EEG microstates were shown to correlate with BOLD activation patterns that resembled the signatures of resting-state networks (Britz et al., 2010; Musso et al., 2010). These findings raise the possibility that the stable and robust patterns described by longtime averages of BOLD fluctuations represent the accumulated effects of much faster, much more dynamic fluctuations in global network states. Much work remains to be done to close the gap between fast and highly variable changes in neural couplings and the slow, coherent and distributed patterns described by large-scale RSNs.

The relation of fast electrophysiological processes and the slow BOLD fluctuations that are measured in resting-state fMRI is further illuminated by MEG studies examining both stationary and nonstationary signal components. MEG recordings of spontaneous brain activity exhibit anatomical patterns that are significantly correlated with those of several fMRI resting-state networks (de Pasquale et al., 2010). Some of these relationships are revealed when taking into account only stationary aspects of the MEG data. However, additional structural features of resting-state networks appear when the nonstationarity aspects of MEG are considered. Broadband MEG power time series show marked non-stationarity, with large power fluctuations that occur on a time scale of seconds. These nonstationarities result in more variable synchronization patterns, with intermittent epochs of high functional coupling that are interspersed by more weakly coherent episodes. These results suggest the possibility that MEG and fMRI recordings probe somewhat different physiological processes reflecting neural synchronization at different levels of variability and robustness.

Even the slow and seemingly stationary signal fluctuations measured by fMRI during cognitive rest now appear more variable and heterogeneous than previously suspected (see, e.g., Smith et al., 2012). Chang and Glover (2010) conducted a detailed analysis of resting-state functional connectivity, including temporal variability of cross-correlations. When they used a sliding window for estimating correlations between neural time series of the posterior cingulate cortex (PCC) and other regions of the brain, significant variations in the strength of these correlations on a time scale of tens of seconds became apparent (figure 6.10). Interestingly, the sliding-window analysis revealed transient correlations of PCC with a set of regions that included not only other regions within the default mode network but also regions that are commonly engaged in attention-demanding task processing.[12] While efforts were made to exclude physi-

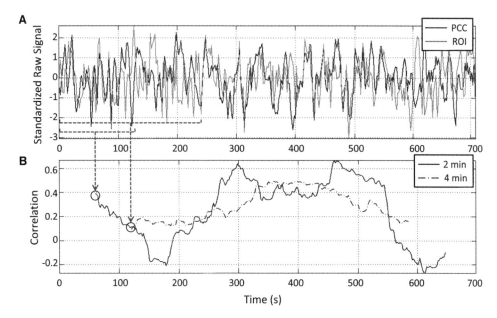

Figure 6.10

Dynamic changes in functional connectivity. Data displayed in both panels are from a single resting functional magnetic resonance imaging scan of a single participant. (A) Blood oxygen level dependent signal fluctuations in posterior cingulate cortex (PCC) and a region of interest (ROI) located in the right inferior frontal operculum (Brodmann area 44). (B) Correlations between the two time courses in (A) for a 2-minute and a 4-minute sliding window. Note that correlations vary greatly in magnitude and even change sign several times during the run. Modified (relabeled and converted to grayscale) and reproduced with permission from Chang and Glover (2010).

ological or motion-induced artifacts, future studies are needed to identify the neural origin for these fMRI nonstationarities. One possible explanation suggests that nonstationary correlations are associated with changes in internal state and cognition. The hypothesis is supported by recent fMRI data on specific patterns of dynamic reconfiguration of functional brain networks in the course of motor learning (Bassett et al., 2011).

It is important to emphasize once again that these nonstationarities and fluctuating patterns of interregional coherence unfold on multiple time scales (from minutes to milliseconds) and all occur within the same structural network described by the connectome. Multiple mechanisms contribute to these fluctuations including the metastable nature of neural dynamics as well as varying patterns of neuromodulation that transiently boost or suppress the efficacy of circuit elements (Brezina, 2010). Thus, an identical structural network can, at different times, support variable functional couplings and interactions. Clearly, this underscores the need for a much more dynamical view of how function emerges from the connectome than is implied by the simplistic view of the connectome as wiring diagram (see chapter 1). This is all the more the case since dynamic variability is increasingly viewed as an important ingredient for flexibility in behavior and cognitive processing.

The rich dynamics of fluctuating functional interactions appear to transcend the narrow bounds imposed by the sparse and rigid skeleton of neuroanatomy. Does this imply that when it comes to understanding these fast dynamic processes the underlying anatomy simply does not matter? Here, an important question to ask is whether different architectures of structural networks are equally capable of fostering rich and variable dynamics. The answer appears to be that certain types of structural brain connectivity create conditions that favor the emergence of rich system dynamics and, thus, flexible computation (see chapter 7). Several architectural features of the human connectome, particularly its hierarchical modularity, play a key role in this process. The emerging picture is one where the architecture of the connectome promotes or enables rich dynamic behavior, rather than acting as a circuit board whose wiring rigidly determines the flow of neural operations.

More Than a Wiring Diagram

The research program of connectomics encompasses not only the tracing and tracking of neural connections at micro-, meso-, and macroscales (see chapters 4 and 5). It must also address the complex problem of how these connections are functionally expressed. As this chapter documented, the connectivity of the human brain powerfully shapes its neural dynamics, the firing patterns of neurons and activations of brain regions. As connectivity shapes dynamics, it is also subject to spontaneous and experience-dependent mechanisms of structural plasticity that constantly rewire and remodel its connection topology (see chapter 3). This dialogue between structure and dynamics is a central feature of many complex networks whose connectivity evolves through time, subject to multiple sources of selection pressure and adaptation. It is important to remember that brain function extends to brain–body–environment interactions, an extended network of relationships through which behavior exerts causative effects on the structure and dynamics of the nervous system. Sensory inputs, and thus their associated brain states, depend on an organism's action in the environment. Thus, in so many ways, understanding the connectome must go beyond the wiring diagram.

This point is significant because it relates to the central issue of how the "connectome in motion" turns brain structure into function. The importance of the connectome partly derives from its role as an intermediate phenotype positioned at the intersection between genetics and environment (figure 6.11). The connectome reflects heritable traits laid down in connectivity, participates in generating behavior, and retains records of an organism's past experience in its biological and social environment. This places the connectome in a central position within a hierarchy of forces that shape an organism's physical form and behavior. This central role is a key motivating factor for studying the connectome in the context of brain and mental disorders, where the clear definition of neurocognitive phenotypes faces numerous difficulties (Congdon et al., 2010). The connectome may offer a new approach

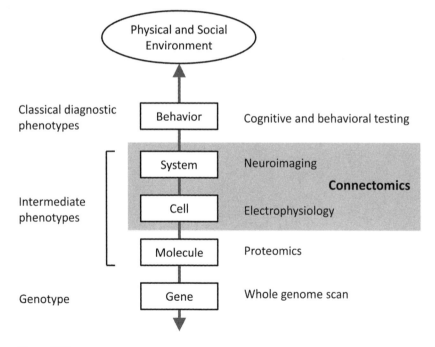

Figure 6.11
The connectome as an intermediate phenotype. This schematic diagram illustrates a hierarchy of brain phenotypes, driven by genetic variation and environmental factors. Connectomics is placed near the center of the hierarchy. Modified after Bullmore et al. (2009).

toward unraveling the genetic bases of disease states of the brain. Alterations of large-scale brain networks have been found to be associated with virtually all neurological or psychiatric conditions studied so far (Menon, 2011). A growing number of studies suggest that many of these disease-related alterations can be traced to structural differences in the spatial layout and topology of the human connectome, reflecting the combined effects of genetic factors, developmental processes, physiology, and environment.[13]

The convergence of genetic and environmental factors onto the structure of the connectome predicts an important role in disease states. It also presents significant new opportunities for collecting comprehensive data on connectivity, behavior, and genetics that can be examined for previously unknown statistical dependencies and regularities. The growing availability of neuroinformatics databases not only promotes innovative new strategies for relating connectivity to brain function but also stimulates the application of network theory (see chapter 7) and the development of integrative brain models (see chapter 8). These new theoretical and computational approaches are beginning to provide a wealth of new insights about the principles that underlie human brain architecture.

7   Emerging Principles of Network Architectures

The characterization of the brain's topological and spatial network architecture is a prime goal of human connectomics (figure 7.1). As connectome-mapping techniques continue to evolve, it is all but inevitable that future technological breakthroughs will substantially enhance our current picture of the network architecture of the human brain. The application of network analysis and modeling tools has already become a core area of computational connectomics by not only offering a variety of tools for data analysis but also providing an important theoretical framework for representing and interpreting connectomes. While our understanding of the network architecture of the human connectome is still incomplete, a number of features of the brain's connection topology and its spatial embedding have been consistently identified (for review, see Bullmore and Sporns, 2009; Sporns, 2011a). Analyses of connectome data include a broad range of local and global network metrics (see chapter 1; Rubinov and Sporns, 2010; Kaiser, 2011). These metrics range from degree distributions, clustering, and path length to the identification of modules and subnetworks, and their hierarchical and spatial embedding. To date, a great majority of studies have used standard anatomical atlases or random partitioning schemes to define network nodes. More recently, parcellation methods developed on the basis of regional differences in cytoarchitectonics, gene expression, and connectivity are beginning to deliver more objective and neurobiologically realistic node definitions (see chapter 5), and thus more accurate network descriptions.

These methodological refinements continue to bring the topological and spatial attributes of the human brain into sharper focus. Here we review some of the major themes that have consistently emerged over recent years. Perhaps the most compelling insights have revealed the human brain as a set of interconnected communities ranging in scale from neurons to brain regions.

A   B

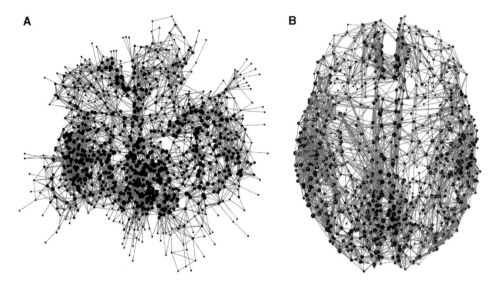

Figure 7.1
Topology and spatial embedding. The two images show the same network of a human brain, a subset of the connections forming its structural backbone as reported in Hagmann et al. (2008). (A) The network is displayed in two dimensions using a topology-based layout algorithm that places nodes and edges in order to minimize a spring-based energy function (Kamada and Kawai, 1989). (B) The same network displayed as a three-dimensional spatially embedded object. Nodes correspond to brain regions and are placed at their anatomical coordinates. Edges are drawn as straight lines between them (see also figure 1.1 for a different example). Data from Hagmann et al. (2008).

Modules and Hubs in the Human Brain

There is a dearth of data describing structural connectivity matrices for cellular networks, and not a single such data set currently exists for any portion of the human brain. This lack of microscale data on human synaptic connectivity is a major rationale for studies conducted in "model systems" from other species. An important ongoing controversy is whether statistical descriptions of cellular connectivity suffice to account for physiological observations (see chapter 3). Since dense reconstructions of neural volumes are still difficult to obtain, most extant connectional data on circuitry come from statistical descriptions of cellular connectivity (Binzegger et al., 2010) or are based on inferences from physiological recordings (Song et al., 2005; Perin et al., 2011) obtained mostly in rodent cortex. Both types of data suggest that cellular connectivity exhibits numerous nonrandom features, including layer- and cell-type-specific as well as distance-dependent connection patterns and specific connection motifs (see also Ganmor et al., 2011). In one of the first studies in this area, Song et al. (2005) simultaneously recorded activity from multiple cells in rat visual cortex and detected several network motifs that were highly overrepresented compared to null models. Synaptic strength appeared to follow a lognormal distribution, indicating the presence of a significant proportion of stronger synapses among mostly weak ones. Interestingly, the density of corticocortical axonal projections determined by tract tracing also follows a broad non-Gaussian (lognormal) distribution (Markov et al., 2011; Wang et al., 2012) suggesting a universal scaling relation across different levels of organization.

Until very recently, virtually no information was available on the degree distributions of different cell types, and data derived from anatomical (as opposed to physiological) observations remain scarce. The average number of synaptic connections (the synaptic degree) for typical cortical neurons is usually estimated to lie between 1,000 and 10,000, but there is a scarcity of data on how this number varies across individual cells belonging to the same morphological class, and hence there is no information on the shape of the degree distribution. A reasonable expectation is that scale-free distributions will likely only exist (if encountered at all) over fairly narrow ranges due to stringent physical limits on synaptic connectivity at the upper end of the scale. This entails that "hub neurons" might derive their centrality primarily from their embedding in the connection topology rather than from their high degree.

A couple of recent reports have added important information regarding cellular circuit topology. In a study involving optical imaging of neurons in developing rodent hippocampus, Bonifazi et al. (2009) demonstrated the existence of functionally highly connected hub neurons in a subpopulation of inhibitory cells. How this high level of functional connectivity relates to underlying structural connection patterns remains to be determined. Most recently, recording activity from up to 12 pyramidal neurons simultaneously, Perin et al. (2011) investigated the topology and synaptic weights among groups of cortical neurons in neonate rat cortex. The study found evidence for nonrandom connectivity that was arranged into a clustered architecture forming a topological small world. Multiple clusters appeared to be interlaced within the same volume of space. The degree distribution of these circuits did not show evidence of scale-free organization, indicating that there were no disproportionately highly connected hub neurons, possibly due to spatial or volume constraints on neuroanatomy. Several statistical relationships between synapse number and density, synaptic weight, and neuronal cluster size could be discerned. Taken together, these studies represent some of the first glimpses of network principles underlying cellular connectivity in a mammalian brain. The emerging picture is one of highly nonrandom organization, with robust statistical patterns for connectivity among neurons and an as yet unknown degree of neuron-to-neuron specificity.

Much more is known about the connection topology of large-scale human brain networks. As reviewed in chapter 5, most structural network analyses of the human connectome are carried out on data acquired with noninvasive diffusion imaging.[1] In most of these studies, primary diffusion imaging and tractography data sets were processed into sparse undirected networks and analyzed with tools from graph theory. Binary network analysis is sometimes carried out by thresholding graded connection information (e.g., Li et al., 2009) or by creating a consensus matrix across a group of participants (e.g., Gong et al., 2009). In weighted network analysis, the edge weights usually represent streamline counts or densities, derived from deterministic tractography. Streamline counts are sometimes taken to be proportional to the magnitude or strengths of axonal tracts linking brain regions (e.g., Hagmann et al., 2008). Other approaches use measurements of the myelination status of pathways to represent connection strength (van den Heuvel et al., 2010; Hagmann et al., 2010b). As noted earlier (see chapter 5), how measures such as numbers of reconstructed fibers or probabilities of fiber tracts relate to neuroanatomy is still far from obvious (Jbabdi and Johansen-Berg, 2011). Tractography infers the probable trajectories of axonal connections, but it does not report directly on their density, magnitude, strength, or direction. Important cross-validation with physiological and anatomical techniques in animal models is urgently needed to better connect imaging constructs to parameters that more directly describe underlying neurobiological structure.

The most fundamental graph measure is the node degree, together with its counterpart in weighted networks, the node strength. Despite the fact that degree and strength are very simple to calculate, there is still some uncertainty regarding the shape of the human connectome's large-scale degree distribution. In good part, this uncertainty is due to the use of variable parcellation methods for node definition.[2] Several studies using random or regional partitions have reported exponential (Hagmann et al., 2008) or exponentially truncated power-law distributions for node degree (Iturria-Medina et al., 2008; Gong et al., 2009; Zalesky et al., 2010). There is general consensus in finding fairly broad degree distributions indicating that brain regions can differ considerably in both node degree and strength. It appears that some regions have considerably stronger and more diverse connection patterns than others.[3]

All human brain network studies published so far have reported the presence of small-world attributes (Bassett and Bullmore, 2006), specifically high clustering and short path length or, equivalently, high local and global efficiency (e.g., Ituria-Medina et al., 2007; Hagmann et al., 2007, 2008; Gong et al., 2009). The coexistence of these two structural characteristics reflects important aspects of network organization, specifically the balance between functional segregation and functional integration which are indexed separately by clustering and path length. Functional segregation ensures that brain regions that are engaged in a common sensory, cognitive, or motor domain can effectively process and share specialized information. High clustering promotes functional segregation because clustered connectivity tends to be concentrated within local network neighborhoods. On the other hand, functional integration ensures that this specialized information can be unified to create coherent brain states and behavioral responses. Short path length or high efficiency indicates that any two nodes in the network can, at least in principle, communicate along fairly direct paths that minimize noise and maximize speed.[4]

It should be noted that small-world attributes provide only very limited information about the network architecture. For example, the original Watts–Strogatz architecture (Watts and Strogatz, 1998) consisted of a regular lattice with a small proportion of randomly rewired edges. However, the organization of large-scale brain networks looks quite different. Connections that are critical for inducing short path length, for example, long-range white matter pathways, have not been added through a process of random rewiring and do not link parts of a uniform lattice. Instead, high clustering in structural brain networks is due to the presence of modules, or local communities of highly and densely connected nodes (Hagmann et al., 2008). These clusters or modules comprise regions that exhibit correlated physiological responses and form coherent functional systems (Hilgetag and Kaiser, 2004). Network elements that belong to the same module often reside within the same volume of space, a design that conserves wiring length as within-module connections tend to be shorter, on average, than between-module connections. Long-distance between-module connections are important for integrating the functionalities of different modules through short paths. Modularity not only is found at the largest scale of whole-brain connectivity but extends to smaller scales as well, an organization that can be described as hierarchical modularity (modules within modules). Modularity at multiple hierarchical scales is found in not only biological but also some electronic information-processing circuits (Bassett et al., 2010; figure 7.2, plate 15) as well as functional brain networks (Meunier et al., 2009).[5]

Degree correlations express the tendency of connected nodes to have a matching number of neighbors. A positive correlation implies that nodes with similar degree tend to be connected while a negative correlation indicates that nodes with dissimilar degree share mutual edges. The metric of assortativity captures this degree correlation across a network (see chapter 1). Many biological networks—for example, protein-interaction networks and food webs—exhibit negative assortativity, indicating that high-degree nodes tend to connect to low-degree nodes and not to each other. Interestingly, the human brain exhibits positive assortativity (Hagmann et al., 2008; Bassett et al., 2010), which is indicative of a tendency for high-degree nodes to connect to other high-degree nodes.[6] High degree is one characteristic of regional hubs, and positive assortativity provides a first indication that high-degree hub nodes are mutually interconnected, forming a hub complex (Sporns et al., 2007), structural core (Hagmann et al., 2008), or a "rich club."

This aggregation of hub nodes is of particular interest in brain networks. In terms of network topology, a rich club is defined as a set of high-degree nodes that forms a tightly interconnected community, often found to play a dominant role in social systems (Colizza et al., 2006). A rich club was first demonstrated in cortical networks of other mammalian species (Zamora-López et al., 2010) where it was found to form a community positioned at the highest level of the connectional hierarchy. More recently, a detailed analysis of the connection topology of the human brain has demonstrated the existence of a rich club of highly connected hub nodes comprising the superior frontal cortex, superior parietal cortex, and the precuneus, in addition to several subcortical regions including the thalamus, hippocampus, and part of the basal ganglia (van den Heuvel and Sporns, 2011; figure 7.3, plate 16). A large fraction of all short paths linking pairs of brain regions pass through the rich club, underscoring its important role in neuronal information transmission and processing. Network models suggest that selective damage to network elements of the rich club has a disproportionate effect on the global efficiency of the remaining network by disrupting numerous long-distance communication paths. Thus, it appears that the human

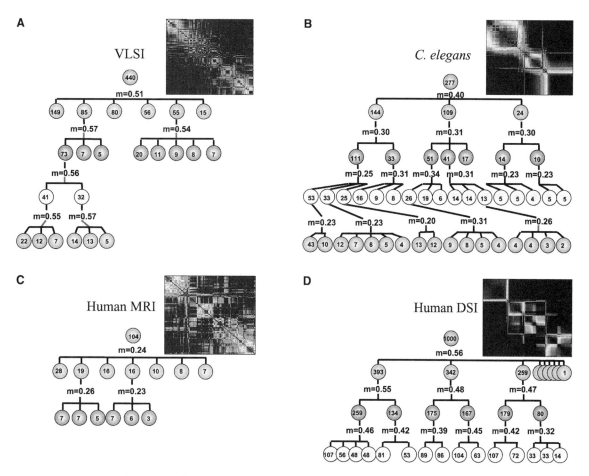

Figure 7.2 (plate 15)
Multiscale modularity in biological and electronic circuits. The four panels show a hierarchical cluster tree of nested modules identified from networks of a very large scale integrated (VLSI) circuit (A), the nematode *C. elegans* (B), a group-averaged anatomical network estimated from structural magnetic resonance imaging (MRI) data of human cerebral cortex (C), and a group-averaged structural network obtained from diffusion spectrum imaging (DSI) and tractography of human cerebral cortex (D). Each branch of the tree shows the breakdown of module sizes and the magnitude of the modularity score *m*. Insets show a color-coded and reordered co-classification matrix expressing, for each node pair, their modular interconnectivity. Reproduced from Bassett et al. (2010a).

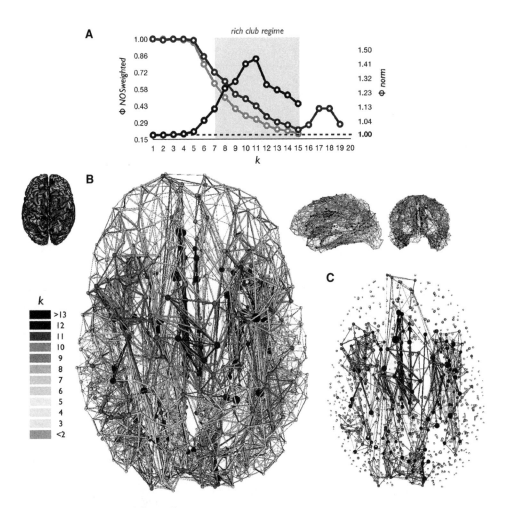

Figure 7.3 (plate 16)
Rich club organization of the human connectome. (A) Plot of the normalized rich-club coefficient φ_{norm} (red curve) against the number of nodes k. At each value of k, all nodes with a degree $<k$ are removed from the network, and the density of connections between the remaining set of nodes (dark gray curve) is evaluated and normalized relative to a random model (light gray curve). A ratio of $\varphi_{norm} > 1$ indicates that the set of k nodes is more highly interconnected than expected by chance. (B) A network diagram for 1,170 randomly partitioned regions of cerebral cortex (nodes) and their interconnections (edges). Color coding (scale at left) indicates the level of participation in the rich club. (C) Same as (B), but only showing the rich-club connections for $k > 9$. Reproduced with permission from van den Heuvel and Sporns (2011).

connectome not only forms a modular small world but also contains a central core of highly and mutually interconnected brain regions. The position of the core or rich club within the connectome's topology predicts a central role for system-wide information flow and integration.

Whether the hub nodes of the human brain are organized in a hierarchy or whether they communicate among each other more "democratically" along uniformly arranged pathways remains to be seen. Multiple lines of evidence support a hierarchical model of hub organization, most of them pointing to the posterior cingulate cortex and adjacent regions of the medial (mesial) parietal cortex, particularly the precuneus, as having a highly central role in structural and functional brain networks. This complex of brain regions is a core component of the default mode network, participating in a large number of functional interactions (Fransson and Marrelec, 2008; Leech et al., 2012). It is activated in a broad range of cognitive tasks, particularly those that involve self-referential processing. Its level of activation or deactivation correlates with the level of consciousness (Laureys et al., 2004), and it exhibits extremely high levels of metabolic activity. Structural analysis of the human connectome has consistently demonstrated not only that the posterior cingulate/precuneus has high centrality (e.g., Hagmann et al., 2008; Gong et al., 2009; van den Heuvel and Sporns, 2011) but also that its position in the network is such that the majority of structural paths that link modules are attached to its core. Interestingly, the high density of cross-hemispheric connections linking core regions across the cerebral hemispheres effectively renders the core a *single* coherent complex. In other words, the topology suggests the existence of an integrated bihemispheric core in medial parietal cortex instead of two separate cores linked by homotopic callosal connections.[7]

Why is the core located in that particular portion of the brain? Part of the explanation may have to do with the fact that the brain is a network that occupies physical space. In such networks, hubs are often found in locations that are not only topologically but also spatially central.[8] Several studies have documented that globally central and highly connected hubs of the human brain aggregate along the cortical midline and are thus positioned between the two cerebral hemispheres in a location that is spatially close to much of the brain. The insula often ranks highly among cortical hubs, and it occupies a spatially central location in each of the two hemispheres (see figure 3.1). Placing hubs in the center of the brain allows them to be reached faster and more efficiently. Recent studies of brain connectivity have begun to focus on this and other aspects of network organization that may have been shaped by the 3D structure of the brain, by its spatial embedding.

Spatial Networks and the Cost-Efficiency Trade-Off

Networks are costly to build and run. The wiring of the physical Internet consumes material resources and energy, as do the transmission lines and transformers of the power grid or the layout of an electronic circuit or computer chip. The cost of these networks principally depends on the spatial placement of their constituent elements. Many social, technological, and natural systems are embedded in space, with nodes and edges taking on specific locations (Barrat et al., 2005; Gastner and Newman, 2006; Barthelemy, 2011). Space is one of the most fundamental factors driving network organization. In many cases, spatial embedding is a key contributor to network cost and performance. For example, spatial embedding can be a decisive factor in determining the location of hub nodes. The topology of transportation networks offers many examples. In airline networks, the topology of connecting flights depends strongly on geographic distances and the distribution of population centers, in addition to community structure reflecting geopolitical constraints (Guimerà et al., 2005). The greater cost of long-distance flights dictates a "hub-and-spoke" organization and generates selection pressure toward locations that offer a combination of low cost and efficient performance. The rise of Dubai as a major international hub can be partially attributed to its geographic location placing it within four hours' flying time of 2 billion people and allowing most large cities on Earth to be linked via Dubai in only one stop.[9] Other examples of spatial embedding that shapes connection topology are found in the physical infrastructure of the Internet's routers and cables (Yook et al., 2002).

The human brain is another example of such a spatial network.[10] Its neural elements and connections occupy specific spatial positions relative to each other. This spatial embedding of nodes and edges is critical as it imposes cost constraints on the network that are reflected in its topology. The growth and maintenance of neural elements and connections consumes metabolic energy, and the neural infrastructure occupies brain volume and imposes conduction delays on neuronal communication (Laughlin and Sejnowski, 2003). It has long been recognized that the design of the nervous system appears to have many features that suggest economical use of limited resources.[11] Cost constraints appear to have shaped topology to a considerable degree, as many network studies have shown that length and volume of neural wiring is highly conserved and near minimal (Chen et al., 2006; Kaiser and Hilgetag, 2006; Rivera-Alba et al., 2011). Wiring length and volume are closely related to the speed with which impulses are conducted and thus influence the timing of neural processing. The spatial embedding of the brain imposes severe upper bounds on how many physical connections a given neuron or brain region can sustain, reflected in high-degree "cutoffs" that are often seen in degree distributions of structural networks. Connections not only consume space and volume but also require large amounts of metabolic energy for signal flow and transmission, in addition to the steady supply of cellular material to sustain the rapid turnover and remodeling of their structural components (see chapter 3). In fact, as noted in chapter 6, the brain's energy demand accounts for a disproportionate amount of the organism's entire energy budget.

However, while the combined cost imposed by energy demand and spatial embedding places stringent constraints on brain architecture and topology, it cannot fully account for all its characteristic features. Some aspects of topology—for example, the propensity for efficient information flow and short path length—can only be achieved if cost constraints are relaxed—for example, by permitting the existence of costly long-distance connection pathways (Kaiser and Hilgetag, 2006). The presence of these pathways promotes the network's capacity to integrate information, but it does so at the expense of energy and volume. This trade-off between cost and efficiency has a powerful influence on human brain connectivity (Bullmore and Sporns, 2012). It may also be the key driving force behind commonalities in topological features observed across multiple natural and artificial information-processing networks. These commonalities include a scaling relation between the number of processing elements and connections that holds for both network topology and spatial embedding (Bassett et al., 2010a).

Is human brain connectivity optimal, either in regard to its computational capacity or its use of material resources? The availability of increasing amounts of connectome data will enable the systematic assessment of "optimality" of brain connectivity, as measured against criteria of metabolic and wiring cost, on the one side, and processing efficiency on the other. Initial indications are that human brain organization reflects a closely negotiated trade-off between cost and efficiency. Computational explorations support this idea. For example, rewiring the human cerebral cortex by randomizing connections not only degrades topological small-world attributes and thus disrupts the balance between segregation and integration but also sharply increases the cost imposed by wiring length (figure 7.4). Random rewiring tends to disrupt modularity and thus degrades one of the most prominent features of brain network architecture that both conserves cost and promotes functional specialization.

A review of the rapidly growing literature on network correlates of brain and mental disorders reveals a tendency for disease conditions to be associated with disturbances of the brain's "high-cost" architectural elements. For example, degenerative conditions such as Alzheimer's disease are accompanied by reduced network efficiency, possibly due to loss of costly long-range connections (Sorg et al., 2007; Stam et al., 2007). The early accumulation of molecules indicative of cell damage and degeneration in central hub regions such as the posterior cingulate cortex/precuneus (Buckner et al., 2009) may be due to the high metabolic cost of connectivity attached to hub nodes, which renders them susceptible to cell damage. A pattern of damage to high-cost network elements is also seen in schizophrenia albeit in different ways. For example, the path lengths of some brain regions, specifically subsets of frontal and temporal regions, were increased, and their centrality was decreased, in structural networks of patients with schizophrenia compared to healthy controls (van den Heuvel et al., 2010), perhaps a result of global reductions in white matter connectivity (Zalesky et al., 2011). Whether these or other clinical conditions are indeed caused by an imbalance in the cost-efficiency trade-off, through developmental or degenerative processes, remains to be seen. If, in fact, high-cost elements like hubs and long-range pathways are centrally responsible for integrative aspects of brain function, even subtle disruptions of their functionality may become manifest in disproportionate disturbances of cognition and behavior.

Finally, the architecture of brain networks must be regarded as the product of development. Numerous aspects of network topology are constrained by molecular and cellular mechanisms of axonal pathfinding and synaptogenesis that favor specific spatial layouts of axonal connections, ranging from genetic "tool kits" and gene regulatory mechanisms to mechanical and tensile forces resulting from differential tissue growth, layering, and folding.[12] These developmental processes mold connectivity patterns and thus leave an imprint on network topology in the adult brain. Physical and developmental constraints rule out a vast set of connection patterns that simply cannot exist as part of a real biological organism, regardless of its evolutionary history, because they cannot be built or sustained (Sporns, 2011a). This observation opens up the

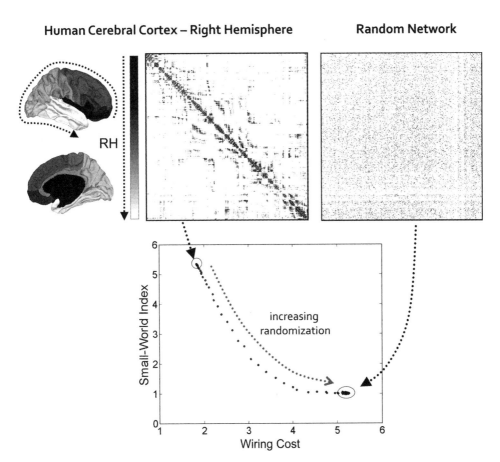

Figure 7.4
Small-world topology and wiring cost in the human cerebral cortex. The figure shows how randomly rewiring the human brain gradually degrades small-world attributes and results in higher wiring cost. The connection matrix at the right corresponds to the right hemisphere (RH) of cerebral cortex, as reported in Hagmann et al. (2008). The matrix consists of 500 patches of cortex, arranged in a frontal–parietal–occipital–temporal ordering. Note that many connections fall along the matrix diagonal, indicating that they are short and connect nearby patches. The matrix at the right is derived from the matrix on the left by fully randomizing the connectivity but preserving node degrees. As randomization proceeds (bottom diagram) the cortical matrix loses its small-world organization. At the same time, its wiring cost, estimated as the total length of all fibers in the brain, more than doubles. Reproduced with permission from Sporns (2011b).

interesting possibility that much about human cognition, to the extent that it depends on the network structure of the connectome, can be explained with reference to the genetic and physical forces that shape brain connectivity in development, subject to the trade-off between network cost and efficiency. Put differently, a combination of factors that per se have little to do with "adaptation for function" or with selection pressure on specific behaviors may have exerted a powerful influence on shaping human cognitive styles and abilities.

While much about the architecture of the connectome remains to be discovered, some consistent themes have already emerged, especially the importance of modularity and hubs for functional specialization and integration. It appears that the cost-efficiency trade-off imposed on the brain by its physical embedding and energy demand drives several major features of brain network organization discerned so far, including its hierarchical modularity as well as its core and rich-club hub-and-spoke architecture. These structural features of the human connectome have important consequences for brain dynamics and for the configuration of functional brain networks.

Functional Networks

In the previous chapter, I discussed at length how functional connectivity, or more generally brain dynamics, emerges from the underlying anatomical pattern of the connectome. A major insight was that variable functional connections give rise to a large repertoire of network states that far transcends the sparse set of couplings comprising a description of the brain's wiring diagram. The size and diversity of this repertoire critically depend on connectome topology. Put differently, given a fixed number of nodes and edges, the way these nodes and edges are interconnected shapes the type of dynamics that can emerge. Neural dynamics, whether measured as sequences of action potentials among individual neurons or as mean firing levels among neuronal populations, give rise to information processing and computation.[13] Neural information processing relies on the capacity of neurons to generate complex probability distributions that represent and encode important features of the internal and external world. Connectivity is absolutely critical for creating and maintaining the informational capacities of neurons and neuronal populations.

As it turns out, not all types of neural dynamics are equally capable of supporting rich information processing. Of particular interest are brain dynamics that exhibit critical behavior (Plenz and Thiagarajan,

2007; Chialvo, 2010), characterized by a mixture of randomness and order, with dynamic transients that ripple across multiple spatial and temporal scales. Theoretical studies suggest that such transients are well suited for flexible computation, and they are thought to be important for information processing in the brain (Beggs, 2008). Transients are also a hallmark of spontaneous and task-evoked brain dynamics, independent of recording method. Which patterns of brain connectivity optimally promote the rich computational capacity associated with critical brain dynamics? Computational studies have demonstrated that key characteristics of critical brain dynamics are strongly associated with specific architectural motifs. Rubinov et al. (2011) investigated this relationship in simulations of ensembles of spiking neurons by varying their connection topology. Hierarchical modularity was found to not only promote low wiring cost but also to broaden a critical regime in neural dynamics, supporting a rich repertoire of population neural activity spanning multiple spatial and temporal scales. Graph-theoretic studies of the human connectome have suggested that hierarchical modularity is indeed one of the hallmarks of brain organization (e.g., Bassett et al., 2010a). The association between dynamic criticality and hierarchical modularity is strongly suggestive of a potential link between connectome topology and the richness of the brain's functional repertoire.

Human brain functional networks share several topological attributes with those of the underlying structural substrate. One example is the shape of degree distributions, which is broad and non-Gaussian for both structural and functional networks. The exact shape of degree distributions of functional brain networks depends in part on the parcellation scheme. Comparing voxel and regional partitions, Hayasaka and Laurienti (2010) found that functional degrees were best modeled by exponentially truncated power laws, with a more pronounced tendency toward power laws at finer partitions. Another example is the tendency of both structural and functional networks to form clusters or modules. Commonly derived by thresholding of strong functional linkages, functional connectivity in the resting brain is organized into communities or modules that correspond to resting-state networks (see chapter 6). These resting-state networks often have components that are spatially distributed and linked by long-distance structural connections.

Another area of considerable interest is the identification of "functional hubs"—brain regions that occupy a central position within functional brain networks. In the earlier discussion of structural hubs we had identified several prominent parts of the cerebral cortex, particularly along the cortical midline, as well as several subcortical regions as widely and centrally connected. Are the same regions exhibiting high centrality in functional brain networks? At first glance, there is indeed some overlap between structural and functional hubs as demonstrated by two studies based on resting-state fMRI. Buckner et al. (2009) identified several core regions of the default mode network as functional hubs in resting-state connectivity, including the posterior cingulate cortex/precuneus, the lateral parietal cortex, and the medial prefrontal cortex. These regions were identified on the basis of node degree, essentially counting the number of strong and positive functional relationships they maintained. Tomasi and Volkow (2010, 2011a, 2011b) used a measure of regional density of functional connections to search for functional hubs and identified a region located in the posterior cingulate cortex/ventral precuneus as the most prominent functional hub in the human brain. This region is virtually identical to the structural core identified with diffusion imaging and tractography (Hagmann et al., 2008).

A caveat in studies of functional networks is the statistical nature of the principal measure, usually a simple linear cross-correlation between time series which, in the case of resting-state fMRI, is sampled over an extended recording period lasting several minutes. The magnitude of these correlations may not have a simple relationship to the true functional centrality of a brain region. For example, a functional hub may be expected to participate in the activity of a diverse set of brain regions and networks, which might increase its dynamic variance and, paradoxically, decrease the longtime average of many of its functional connections. Thus, the "functional centrality" of a neural hub may be difficult to assess. To further investigate this issue, Zuo et al. (2012) conducted a systematic comparison of several network centrality measures applied to resting-state fMRI. These measures included degree, subgraph centrality (Estrada and Rodriguez-Velázquez, 2005), eigenvector centrality (Bonacich, 1972), and page-rank centrality (Page et al., 1999). The two latter measures express centrality not only on the basis of local node properties but recursively take into account the centrality of connected nodes. Zuo et al. (2012) found that each measure disclosed different aspects of "functional centrality" and suggested that a combination of several different centrality measures might be useful for charting different aspects of information flow in the human functional connectome.

The search for "functional hubs" illustrates some of the caveats that must be taken into account when comparing graph measures in structural and functional networks. The interpretation of connection topology in functional connectivity requires careful consideration of the neurobiological meaning of nodes and edges (Rubinov and Sporns, 2010). For example, anatomical interpretations of MEG or EEG recordings are made difficult because of the nonlocal nature of the recorded electromagnetic fields while networks derived from fMRI time series cross-correlations necessarily include many couplings along indirect structural paths (see chapter 6). Furthermore, functional networks are increasingly viewed as evolving across time, with rapid changes in connectivity that reflect nonstationary neural dynamics (e.g., Smith et al., 2012). These and other considerations strongly suggest that despite some commonalities in topology, structural and functional brain networks must be carefully distinguished from one another when it comes to analysis and interpretation. Future studies of their relationship will benefit from more advanced methodology—for example, in the area of effective (or causal) connectivity.

These methodological developments are particularly important since functional connectivity, particularly longtime averages of resting-state BOLD signal fluctuations, are widely studied in the context of disease states. Virtually all brain and mental disorders have been found to be associated with specific disturbances of functional connectivity. In some disorders, like schizophrenia, theories of "disconnection" have a long history extending over more than a century. Network analysis of connectome data represents a new and promising approach toward understanding how cognitive and behavioral deficits originate from disruptions of network connectivity and information flow (Bassett and Bullmore, 2009; Guye et al., 2010; Zhang and Raichle, 2010). Network analysis can sensitively capture individual variations of network topology in relation to cognitive capacity in healthy participants (e.g., van den Heuvel et al., 2009b; Bassett et al., 2009; Li et al., 2009). These variations then provide connectivity phenotypes that can be investigated in the context of individual experience, development, and genetic background, possibly yielding novel biomarkers for brain and mental disorders. Noninvasive MR connectomics has already provided new insights into changes in network organization associated with mental diseases such as schizophrenia (Bassett et al., 2008; Skudlarski et al., 2010; van den Heuvel et al., 2010; Zalesky et al., 2011). Studies of structural and functional networks in schizophrenia are beginning to converge on identifying globally disturbed network topology that results from deficits in specific hub nodes and cortical pathways. Future studies will likely combine graph analysis with heritability and genomic data to disentangle genetic and environmental influences on connectome topology. Harnessing the full potential of connectomics for understanding disease states will require new methods for quantitative comparison of connectomes across individuals and control/patient populations.

What's Human about the Human Connectome?

Early studies of connection maps, mostly acquired through noninvasive diffusion imaging and tractography, are beginning to reveal key attributes of human brain network organization. Among these attributes is a pronounced community structure with modules that are hierarchically arranged and interconnected through a core complex or rich club of hub nodes. The connectome is arranged economically, conserving structural and metabolic cost, while also performing efficiently by ensuring direct and global information flow. The origin of this cost-efficiency trade-off lies in the spatial embedding of the human brain, in its physical realization as a collective of cells and circuits that consume space and energy.

Do these early studies allow us to pinpoint any features of network organization that are specifically human? Are there any aspects of connection topology or complexity that set the human brain apart from those of other species? At the time of writing, the answer to this question is unknown.[14] Comparative analyses point to many aspects of network organization that are common among a range of biological nervous systems, even including technological information-processing systems such as electronic circuits (Bassett et al., 2010a). At least some of these commonalities may be explained on the basis of shared selection pressures that relate to the trade-off between cost and efficiency that must be negotiated by all information-processing networks. Other features of the human connectome may yet turn out to be, if not unique to humans, then perhaps more highly expressed in the human brain compared to that of other species. For example, the aggregation of hub nodes into a rich club (van den Heuvel and Sporns, 2011) and the elaboration of a subset of long-range pathways related to specifically human cognitive capacities such as language (Catani et al., 2005) are good candidates for important structural substrates of integrative cognitive processes. It may also be important to look beyond the confines of the brain itself. Perhaps some of our uniquely human cognitive capacities are not a simple function of the number of neurons and synapses, or even their networked interactions, and instead are better understood as the product of how our brains are acting in and on our increasingly complex social and cultural environments.

We still know very little about the evolution of brain networks. Ongoing and future studies promise significant new insights in this regard, for example by way of assembling comprehensive connectome maps across a range of vertebrate and invertebrate species. As connectomics technology continues to mature, the cost and effort needed to extract a given brain's connection pattern is likely to fall considerably. A worthwhile albeit distant goal is the collection and comparison of connectivity maps from a broad range of species in order to identify their commonalities and differences.[15] A catalog of connectomes would allow identifying relations between brain architecture and body plans, developmental mechanisms, behavioral capacities, and cognition. Such a catalog could lay a foundation for "comparative connectomics" and provide clues about potential evolutionary trends in brain connectivity. A promising target of investigation is the evolution of modularity. Based on current knowledge, it appears that structural modules and small-world attributes are found in both invertebrate (e.g., Chiang et al., 2011) and vertebrate species, but it is not known if modularity increases with species complexity or how it relates to scaling laws—for example, the relation of gray and white matter volume in mammalian brains (Zhang and Sejnowski, 2000) or the number of anatomically distinct brain regions (Krubitzer, 2007).

Extracting principles of brain architecture is a major goal of connectomics, not only because it provides insight into brain organization, including its developmental and evolutionary origins, but also because such principles are key ingredients of computational models of brain function. Such models play an increasing role in neuroscience, and as connectomics matures, we may expect to see a new generation of such models emerge—models of "virtual brains." The final chapter explores the current status and future growth of computational connectomics.

The complementarity of structure–function relations in the brain, the parallel existence of multiple spatial and temporal scales, and the sheer size of connectome data sets make computational approaches to modeling and data analysis essential and indispensable. While some modeling and analysis can proceed by way of heuristics, deeper explorations of the human connectome must be guided by the theoretical framework of network science. As discussed at length in the previous chapter, network approaches provide far more than just capable and versatile data analysis methods. They also establish a link between brain connectivity, on the one side, and the considerable body of theory on complex networks on the other. This final chapter is about the rapidly expanding role of informatics and computation in analysis and modeling of connectome data, including the use of network models for creating computer simulations of the human brain.

The arrival of connectome data sets has already opened up new possibilities for computational modeling in neuroscience. Network models of the connectome have begun to reveal architectural principles that enable the brain's computational efficiency and flexibility. For the first time, empirically measured whole-brain connectivity matrices have been employed in large-scale simulations of neural dynamics, a step toward constructing comprehensive mechanistic models of the human brain. Such models are important because, as we discussed earlier, the connectome does not translate into functional connectivity or, for that matter, into cognition and behavior in ways that can simply be read out from the connection topology. Instead, models are needed to both explain and predict system behavior. Such models offer much more than tools for describing empirical data or for performing statistical inferences on hypotheses. They are essential for uncovering causal and generative mechanisms underlying neural and behavioral observations (Breakspear and McIntosh, 2011). One of the main motivating forces at the origin of connectomics was the creation of whole-brain models whose dynamics match empirical neural recordings and that can give rise to realistic behavior (Sporns, 2012). The availability of connectome data sets now allows the construction of such virtual brain models that can be tested against empirical data.

This chapter surveys the prospects for developing realistic computational models of the human brain that can aid basic and applied research and provide an objective way to organize our knowledge about human cognition. But first, we turn to the considerable challenge posed by cataloguing and disseminating the growing amount of human connectome data.

Neuroinformatics Challenges

In 1989 nanotechnology and cryonics expert Ralph Merkle wrote a remarkably prescient technical report for Xerox Corporation, in which he predicted that "a complete analysis of the cellular connectivity of a structure as large as the human brain is only a few decades away" (Merkle, 1989, p. 1). Merkle sketched out an approach to imaging the structure of the human brain at subcellular resolution quite similar to EM strategies that are currently pursued in microscale connectomics (see chapter 4). He realized that carrying out such a project would require automated reconstruction and storage of very large data sets—so large in fact that the computational resources available at the time were far outmatched. Assuming around 10^{24} elementary computational operations for imaging and reconstruction, and given the cost of computing around 1990, Merkle's estimate for the total price tag of the project came to 34 billion dollars, a number he expected to drop to 34 million dollars over the following 20 years.[1]

Clearly, estimates for the size of data sets and the computational effort involved in reconstruction and analysis depend on the scale at which data are acquired. On the microscale of EM and LM approaches, the raw data for a structure the size of the human brain would require a zettabyte (a trillion gigabytes) of memory, currently beyond the storage capacity of any computer (Kasthuri and Lichtman, 2010).[2] On the other hand, connectome data sets obtained at the macroscale with noninvasive imaging technology are large but manageable. For example, the connectomes of 1,200 participants acquired as part of the Human Connectome Project will consume around a petabyte (a million gigabytes) of

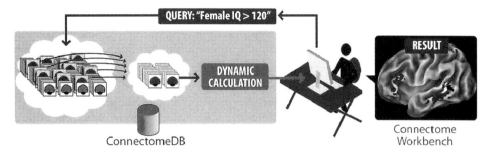

Figure 8.1
Data mining and visualizing the human connectome. Shown here is a schematic example utilizing the tool set envisioned for the National Institutes of Health–funded Human Connectome Project. Connectome data sets can be queried, metrics of interest can be computed from selected subsets, and results can be visualized and rendered graphically. DB, database. Modified (converted to grayscale) and reproduced with permission from Akil et al. (2011).

online storage (Akil et al., 2011). Importantly, the size of raw data sets acquired in microscopy or imaging can be effectively reduced by rendering connectomes in the much more compact form of network descriptions. For example, a connection matrix of a single human brain at the level of millimeter-size voxels would at most require a few gigabytes of memory.

Going beyond data size and storage, additional challenges involve creating data structures that can accommodate different recording methods and modalities, as well as providing resources for users who wish to mine and visualize data sets (figure 8.1). Data types include volume- and surface-based representations of the brain that assign a set of spatial coordinates to each voxel. These coordinates (or "brainordinates"; Marcus et al., 2011) can then be mapped to rows and/or columns of connectivity matrices comprising a separate connectivity-based data type. Jointly, locations in the brain and their mutual associations can be stored, visualized, and processed with a variety of software and rendering tools. Additional neuroinformatics challenges for connectomics involve linking connectivity data to other domains that record individual characteristics of participants, such as data on demographics, behavior, cognitive performance, or genomics.

Several visualization platforms for connectomics are currently under development. These tools allow for interactive queries of specific brain regions or pathways and display data on brain volumes, surfaces, or in network format. The Connectome Workbench, currently under development (Marcus et al., 2011), will be closely linked to a database called ConnectomeDB which will house data from the Human Connectome Project (http://www.humanconnectome.org). Visualization options include fMRI activation data, regional parcellations, contours between cortical areas or parcels, connectivity profiles (essentially the rows/columns of connection matrices projected back into anatomical space), and network metrics computed for specific locations in the brain, as well as time series data in graphical or movie format. Connectivity profiles can be rendered for direct as well as indirect connections. Data can be visualized for individual participants or as group-averaged representations for participant groups selected according to user-supplied criteria. Interactive exploration will include multimodal comparisons, such as between structural and functional connectivity data. Another online software platform, the Connectome Viewer (Gerhard et al., 2011; http://www.connectomics.org/viewer) is more specifically geared toward analysis and visualization of structural connectivity data sets, with numerous options for displaying brain surfaces, fiber trajectories, and distributions of network metrics. Connectome visualization platforms will also allow for the export of brain connectivity data to more generic network analysis tool sets.[3]

Very little progress has been made to date in merging or cross-referencing of connectome data across scales—for example, relating connection data from networks at cellular resolution to large-scale projections and pathways. In part, this is due to the relative paucity of cellular network data, particularly in human brain. The development of multimodal registration tools and connectivity-based data formats for diffusion and functional MRI provides a potential model for future integration efforts across scales. These efforts will be facilitated by the use of network theory, which relies on the universal mathematical structure of graphs, defined as sets of nodes and edges. Graphs can capture connectivity at any scale and thus naturally encompass multiscale architectures and nested connectivity patterns. Future connectome databases may not only provide multimodal linkage at single scales but also allow users to "zoom in" on details of cellular connectivity from large-scale maps, not unlike what is currently possible in Google Earth. For human connectomics, the feasibility of a multiscale connectome database requires the availability of at least some regional volumes for which connectivity is resolved at the microscale. To render the data interpretable to the human user, significant data reduction into network form will be essential.

The future success of connectomics will depend on broad availability of data in open-access repositories and archives.[4] This will allow researchers to gain access to normative data sets, explore and mine data for statistical patterns, and use these data to inform computational models bridging levels of analysis. A major driving force behind efforts to collect and share large data sets is the growing realization that understanding the complexities of brain and behavior requires the integration of scientific findings across a broad array of methods, approaches, and systems (Akil et al., 2011). Whether it is normal behavior and cognition, or disease states, a full understanding is only possible if genetic, neural, and behavioral data are combined and analyzed in context. The creation of open-access large biological data sets enables discovery science, thus complementing more conventional focused and hypothesis-driven research. Progress in this direction will come not only from large, centrally funded research consortia but also from community-driven "grassroots" initiatives.[5] Biswal et al. (2010) spearheaded efforts to create a public repository for resting-state fMRI combining data sets of 1,414 participants independently collected at more than 30 globally distributed MR centers. This 1000 Functional Connectomes Project (http://fcon_1000.projects.nitrc.org/) was made possible not only by an unprecedented degree of global collaboration among researchers but also by the adoption of a connectomics framework, which allowed representation of these data with the common "language" of connectivity and networks.[6] These data have already been widely used by a number of researchers and have led to new insights about universal and individual features of brain organization (e.g., community structure and hub regions; Tomasi and Volkow, 2010, 2011a, 2011b; Rubinov and Sporns, 2011; Zuo et al., 2012).

It is likely that interest in connectome data will further increase as a growing number of studies disclose relations between brain connectivity and genetic markers (see below). Atlas-based comparisons between gene expression and connectivity have already been carried out in rodents (French and Pavlidis, 2011; French et al., 2011; Wolf et al., 2011) and will soon become possible in the human brain as well, as online databases on gene expression in the human brain[7] become cross-referenced with human connectome data. For example, spatially registered bidirectional links between the Allen Human Brain Atlas and the Human Connectome Project will allow users of both databases to access genomic or connectivity data for specific anatomic locations (Marcus et al., 2011).

Neuroinformatics efforts benefit from the adoption of a common format for how connectome data are represented. The sheer size and volume of primary data sets from EM/LM or neuroimaging is a major challenge for effective data sharing. The reduction of these data to structural and functional networks not only is economical but greatly facilitates comparison and interpretation, and it enables the use of a broad range of network analysis and modeling approaches.

Building a Virtual Brain

Complex systems cannot be fully understood without the use of computational models that simulate system dynamics and allow prediction of future behavior following perturbation. Such computational models typically build on an understanding of the basic elements and interactions that are relevant for global system behavior. In physics, computational models are deployed over an astounding range of systems, all the way from the dynamics of single molecules to the motions of galaxies. In the social sciences, the increasing availability of massive amounts of data through digital communication, financial and economic monitoring, and social media has led to a surge in the creation of quantitative data-driven models of social systems (Lazer et al., 2009).[8] In computational biology, significant efforts have been directed at designing models of cells that allow an understanding of how their molecular components work together to generate global functional states. The cell biologist Masaru Tomita suggested that the "study of the cell will never be complete unless its dynamic behavior is understood" (Tomita, 2001, p. 205). He argues that dynamic behavior of the cell is more than an inventory of all the parts and goes beyond a static flowchart of chemical reactions and pathways. Accurate prediction requires simulation of system dynamics, setting in motion parts and pathways.

Computational models are becoming an integral part of neuroscience, and connectomics contributes to this trend through fostering the development of connectivity-based models of neural dynamics and behavior. This type of model instantiates specific hypotheses about the causes and mechanisms that generate observed data on neural responses. The process of model building and testing can be visualized as proceeding in two main directions (Valdes-Sosa et al., 2011; figure 8.2). Model-driven approaches instantiate a neural model specified by a set of state equations describing, for example, membrane conductances or mean firing levels, as well as a connection matrix determining the model's synaptic

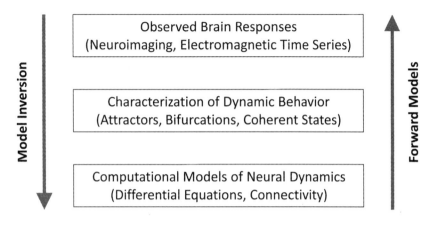

Figure 8.2
Forward models and model inversion. Forward modeling involves computational models
that instantiate biophysical mechanisms and structural connectivity (bottom) and give rise
to organized neural dynamics (middle) that can be compared to empirically observed brain
responses (top). Model inversion involves the objective inference of models that best
explain observed data and can account for important features of brain dynamics. Based on
a similar diagram in Valdes-Sosa et al. (2011).

coupling. The purpose of the model is to explain and predict dynamic
behavior, in the process testing the hypothesis that the form and parameters of the model can account for empirical observations. In contrast,
data-driven approaches start from observations and then attempt to fit
models to the observed data. These models are generative and causal in
that they instantiate neural processes and effective connectivity that
jointly account for the empirical observations. A large number of causal
models are tested, and rigorous model selection criteria are then used to
evaluate the evidence provided by each candidate model. It is important
to realize that both models and empirical observations are subject to
revision and expansion—hence a "final model" of brain function is
unlikely to be achieved in the near (or even distant) future. Rather,
model building and empirical testing is part of an ongoing iterative dialogue between model-driven ("forward modeling") and data-driven
("model inversion") approaches.

System identification is an important part of control theory where it
refers to the inference of dynamical models on the basis of observed data.

For example, fluctuations in economic measures in relation to external perturbations may be used to specify a dynamic model that relates inputs to observations. If there is some knowledge about the mechanisms that underlie system behavior, system identification may be used to infer the parameter distribution of a generative model that can best explain observed responses. In cognitive neuroscience, the framework of dynamic causal modeling (DCM; Friston et al., 2003; Penny et al., 2004) allows not only the comparison of competing hypotheses, implemented as network models, about the neural causes for observed dynamic responses, but also the identification of a network model that best explains data through a process of "network discovery" (Friston et al., 2011). In principle, given the observations and a formally specified generative model, a large model space can be constructed within which DCM, using Bayesian model selection, identifies the model that best explains the data. Critically, DCM compares dynamic models that describe different sets of causal relations specified as directed graphs whereas comparisons of functional connectivity can only yield correlational information without access to underlying neural causes. A current drawback of DCM for network discovery is that it can only be applied to fairly small sets of nodes and edges due to combinatorial explosion of the model space. Here, the incorporation of connectome data could provide strong additional priors that help to constrain the space over which models need to be compared.

Forward models of neural dynamics based on connectome data sets have been used to explain the neural basis of spatiotemporal patterns in spontaneous neural activity—for example, those seen in the brain's resting-state (see chapter 6). A comparative analysis of several computational models (Honey et al., 2007, 2009; Ghosh et al., 2008; Deco et al., 2009) has identified an overall modeling framework that can account for a large body of empirical data (Deco et al., 2011). Three main concepts contribute to this framework: Resting-state dynamics is constrained by the underlying structural connectivity, depends on variable time delays for signal transmission between proximal or remote brain regions, and arises from local interactions among populations of neurons within each region. Jointly, connection topology, conduction delays, and local dynamics give rise to a rich set of functional networks.

Implemented on the connection matrix of a large part of the macaque cortex, a model of coupled chaotic oscillators first demonstrated the dependence of coherent BOLD signal fluctuations on structural connectivity (Honey et al., 2007). Slow changes in BOLD signals were driven by variations in fast synchronization among neural elements that, in turn, are shaped by the structural coupling matrix. Longtime averages of BOLD responses showed significant correspondence between structural and functional connectivity, but at shorter time scales the model exhibited series of transients with variable functional couplings, thus predicting nonstationarities of the type that were later discovered in empirical data (e.g., Chang and Glover, 2010; see figure 6.10). A recent analysis of spontaneous BOLD fluctuations recorded in the macaque monkey and processed into a functional network demonstrated significant agreement between model and empirical data (Adachi et al., 2012; figure 8.3). The model was later expanded to simulate human resting-state functional connectivity. The structural coupling matrix was a weighted representation of anatomical connectivity inferred from diffusion imaging and tractography (Hagmann et al., 2008). The model was able to generate dynamics that closely matched empirically recorded resting-state functional connectivity (Honey et al., 2009). It could also reproduce effects on functional connectivity due to perturbations of specific pathways—for example, the disruption of interhemispheric couplings following callosotomy (Johnston et al., 2008; see figure 6.5).

The model of resting-state dynamics by Ghosh et al. (2008) was also based on a network of anatomical couplings but in addition to the network topology also included conduction delays, thus incorporating the full spatiotemporal coupling matrix, as well as noise. Noise drove the system away from dynamic equilibrium, and subsequent relaxation of model dynamics back toward the stable regime generated series of dynamic transients. The temporal succession of these transients created fluctuations that resembled the brain's resting state. This noise-driven exploration of the neighborhood around the equilibrium state was most pronounced if the system was poised at or near the onset of spontaneous oscillations. The model by Deco et al. (2009) suggested that noise-driven transitions between dynamically multistable states give rise to fluctuations in synchronization patterns which, in turn, drive slow BOLD fluctuations. Connection topology as well as conduction delays were important model ingredients that determine the spatiotemporal patterning of resting-state neural activity. A related model comprising coupled oscillators that engage in time-delayed network interactions showed the emergence of slow fluctuations in neural activity that were related to concomitant BOLD functional connectivity (Cabral et al., 2011). Despite the simplicity of the basic oscillator, the topology and time delays incorporated into the structural connectivity were found to induce patterns of

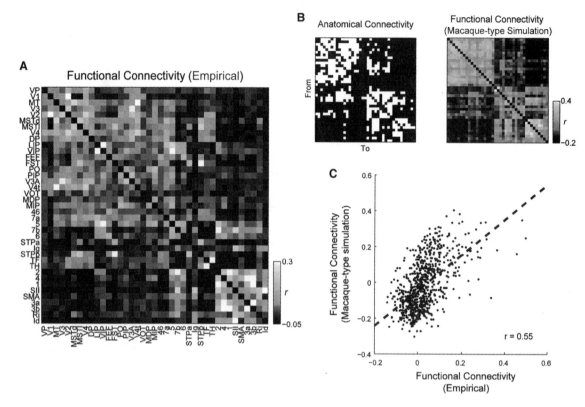

Figure 8.3
Empirical and modeled blood oxygen level dependent (BOLD) functional connectivity in the macaque cortex. (A) A functional connectivity matrix computed from functional magnetic resonance imaging recordings of spontaneous BOLD signals in two anesthetized macaque monkeys. The cortex was parcellated into 39 regions (please see original publication). (B) The anatomical connectivity was derived from published tract-tracing data collated in the CoCoMac database (see chapter 5). The functional connectivity was computed using a neural mass model and simulated BOLD mechanism as reported in Honey et al. (2007). (C) The scatter plot of simulated versus functional connectivity reveals a statistically highly significant correlation of r = 0.55. Modified (converted to grayscale) and reproduced with permission from Adachi et al. (2012).

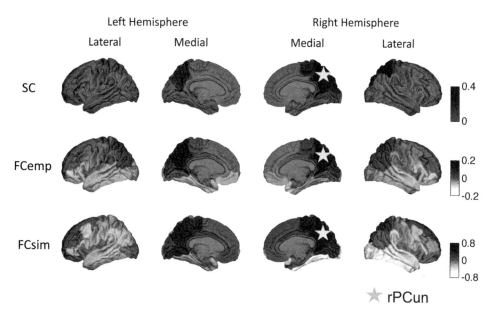

Figure 8.4 (plate 17)
A model of whole-brain dynamics based on coupled oscillators. The figure shows a comparison of structural connectivity (SC), empirically measured functional connectivity (FCemp), and simulated functional connectivity (FCsim), rendered on a standard surface map of the cerebral cortex after seeding from the precuneus in the right hemisphere (rPCun, light blue star). Connectivity patterns are highly correlated, not only between the empirical SC and FCemp (as discussed in chapter 6) but also between FCemp and FCsim, suggesting that the computational model can reproduce many of the anatomical details of functional connectivity. Modified and reproduced with permission from Cabral et al. (2011).

simulated functional connectivity that matched those seen in empirical recordings (figure 8.4, plate 17).

Several insights can be gained from these modeling efforts. All three models reinforce the notion that the connectome shapes spontaneous brain dynamics. As discussed in chapter 6, a growing body of empirical evidence also supports this important idea. However, the models also clearly illustrate some significant limitations. While anatomy can be said to "shape" or "constrain" functional connectivity, even a fixed and unchanging anatomical "skeleton" can give rise to a large number of time-varying patterns of dynamic interactions. This set of patterns can be conceptualized as a "dynamic repertoire" that is continually rehearsed in the resting brain (see chapter 6). Enabling these fluctuations is the proximity of the system to a marginally stable critical dynamic regime. Being close to instability ensures that system dynamics neither die out nor become completely random. As a result, functional connectivity is not a static pattern—it is a series of patterns that emerge from the continual flow of neural dynamics through the state space of the brain. The connectome, through its topology and spatial embedding (as expressed in conduction delays), shapes this flow by creating a dynamic manifold, a low-dimensional subset of brain states that appear as coherent functional units in the resting and working brain. Over longer time scales, these brain states can in turn modify and mold the anatomical linkages of the connectome through mechanisms of activity-dependent plasticity.

It is worth noting that nonstationarities in BOLD fluctuations (see chapter 6; figure 6.10) were first predicted by these models and have only recently come under closer empirical scrutiny. Future applications of the modeling approach involve the construction of a "Virtual Brain" to model human neural dynamics (Jirsa et al., 2010; http://thevirtualbrain .org). Building on empirical data, including data coming from connectome-mapping studies, the goal is to create detailed models that can generate neuronal time series matching those obtained from neuroimaging experiments. The Virtual Brain will allow for the implementation of different formulations of neural population dynamics, and its connectivity structure can come from either group-averaged or individual connectome data sets. The models will include realistic conduction delays and will be explicitly embedded in 3D space, allowing results to be displayed in brain volumes and surfaces. Models can be tested against empirical observations, and they can be subjected to systematic perturbations to evaluate model responses, explicitly in the context of clinical applications. Particularly important will be to devise perturbations that replicate disease processes or the effects of focal brain lesions (e.g., Alstott et al., 2009). The Virtual Brain thus becomes a test bed for exploring disease-related disturbances of the connectome and their dynamic manifestations, opening up new possibilities for developing diagnostic and therapeutic strategies. A future goal is to create patient-specific brain models that build on the individual's connectome and brain geometry to allow the assessment of the dynamic consequences of disease or injury and the prediction of successful intervention and rehabilitation.

Other efforts to build working models of mammalian or human brains are under way, and connectome data will be critical for steering these models toward realistic performance. Dharmendra Modha and colleagues have created an extremely large simulation of a neural model incorporating neuronal spiking dynamics, plasticity, and axonal conduction delays, altogether comprising on the order of 1 billion neurons and 10 trillion synapses (Ananthanarayanan et al., 2009).[9] The size of the model is on the same scale as the cerebral cortex of the cat, and continued improvements in efficient implementation and supercomputing resources may soon allow the model to be run in near-real time. A critical ingredient for generating a model of the cat cortex that resembles its biological counterpart is the cat connectome. Ananthanarayanan et al. implemented probabilistic data on connectivity of local circuits of cat cortex derived from reconstructions of individual neurons (Binzegger et al., 2004). Additional steps toward constructing a working model of the brain will involve the incorporation of interregional projections and of the cerebellum and subcortical regions such as the thalamus.[10] An even greater amount of detail, in particular with respect to cellular morphology and synaptic physiology, is incorporated into Henry Markram's Blue Brain architecture (Markram, 2006. One of the initial project goals is the creation of a realistic simulation of a cortical column, based on data from the rat somatosensory cortex, later to be expanded to a full-sized model of a whole brain.

What do these attempts at modeling complex brains have in common, and how do they differ from each other? Markram's Blue Brain as well as Modha's model of cat cortex aim at simulating the brain at cellular resolution, from the "bottom up," by aggregating cells into circuits, and circuits into neural systems. Modha's model, at the current stage, provides an "existence proof" demonstrating the feasibility of simulating a brain-size model in near real-time on a supercomputer. Markram's model more explicitly aims at generating data that can be related to neurobiological experimentation and guide empirical brain research. An important next step will be for these models to generate specific results that can explain or predict empirical knowledge about cells, circuits, or whole-brain dynamics. So far, neither model has made significant contact with empirical research on human brain anatomy or physiology, despite widely publicized claims that the ultimate goal is to simulate the functioning of the human brain and human cognition.[11] Is ultimate success in this area simply a matter of computational resources, of waiting until Moore's law makes real-time simulations of large brains at cellular or subcellular resolution technologically feasible?

The task of building a truly functional model of the human brain from individual neurons is similar to that of creating models of complex cellular processes by simulating the cell's molecular components, one at a time. However, a successful outcome of such ambitious projects critically depends on knowledge about the organization of neurons and molecules into complex networks whose function underpins system dynamics. A fundamental difficulty facing the bottom-up approach to brain modeling is that it tends to neglect the multiscale nature of brain connectivity and the complex role of connectivity in generating neural dynamics and function. Rather than designing an architecture that incorporates patterns from all scales that are experimentally accessible, including the large scale of neural populations and brain regions, bottom-up approaches attempt to construct the brain by brute force, neuron by neuron and synapse by synapse. What is lacking are the important constraints provided by empirical and theoretical research on principles of brain organization and architecture. Essentially, such bottom-up models perpetuate the Laplacian dream of nineteenth-century physics, encapsulated in the belief that the future of the universe (including brain states) can be fully predicted once the positions and velocities of all elementary particles (neurons and synapses) are known. The point of building brain models, however, is to advance understanding of brain function, not creating in silico replicas that are as complex and incomprehensible as the real thing.

In contrast, the Virtual Brain and related modeling efforts explicitly build on a multiscale, or at least "multiscale-minded," theoretical framework (figure 8.5). This framework recognizes that dynamics at different scales are mutually interdependent across hierarchies of space and time. Multiscale approaches are widely adopted in the physical sciences where they have been extremely successful in areas such as fluid dynamics, magnetization, climatology, materials engineering, and seismicity. Multiscale organization is also a hallmark of many complex networks (see chapter 1), including those found in power systems, the Internet, transportation, epidemiology, and genomic and cellular regulation. What is common to all multiscale approaches is that "scaling up" of system dynamics is not attempted by brute force, involving the explicit simulation of all particles and their interactions. For example, models of fluid dynamics are simply infeasible if all that is allowed are water molecules and their motions. Instead, multiscale approaches embrace models for dimension reduction where processes at smaller scales become part of compact descriptions of regularities at larger scales. Small-scale processes are not "averaged away"—rather, they become part of and contribute to the reduced parameterized description of what the system does as a whole. Computational explorations can iterate between scales, searching for important small-scale mechanisms that have to be incorporated into larger-scale descriptions to afford greater realism. No

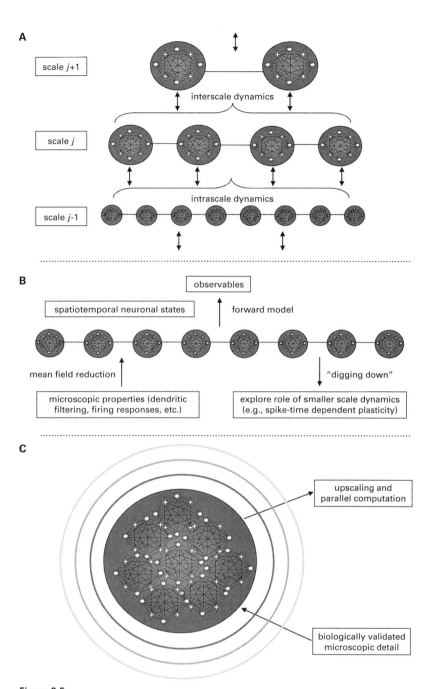

Figure 8.5
Multiscale modeling. Schematic illustration of three different modeling approaches to address the brain's multiscale organization. (A) An explicitly multiscale framework that combines and integrates dynamic models at several scales. (B) A "multiscale-minded" approach that models dynamics explicitly at only one scale but attempts to incorporate mechanisms that reside at smaller scales and to predict dynamics at larger scales (see figure 8.2). (C) A "brute-force" approach working by aggregating dynamics of microscale processes without explicit consideration of how these processes are organized across scales. Redrawn from a similar figure in Jirsa et al. (2010).

single scale is privileged—all scales contribute to macroscopic system behavior.

Multiscale models of brain dynamics are of critical importance for achieving a principled understanding of how neural substrates give rise to behavior and cognition. Such models give rise to a dimensionally reduced set of dynamic patterns that are shaped and constrained by brain connectivity. A major goal for connectomics will be to discern how these patterns are related to the architecture of human cognition.

New Ontology for Human Cognition

In the present context, the term "ontology" refers to a way to organize information about a specific knowledge domain, a structured knowledge base designed to facilitate information sharing. Ontology represents distinct entities or categories within the domain and specifies their properties and relations. Such categorization only makes sense if members of different categories can be distinguished along meaningful dimensions of variance. Thus, finding a suitable ontology requires the identification of the main dimensions of variance that best represent the domain in question. Ontology is an extremely useful tool for organizing large data sets (e.g., gene ontologies; Ashburner et al., 2000; Bard and Rhee, 2004) and for building conceptual maps that relate, explain, and predict research findings. Regarding the human mind, defining a classification scheme or ontology of mental processes has remained an unfulfilled challenge. Psychologists and cognitive scientists continue to rely, for the most part, on an ontology that largely derives from schemes and distinctions drawn decades if not centuries ago. Can connectomics help to find a more principled map for the relations among categories of human mental processing by grounding these categories in the brain's network architecture?

Traditionally, mappings between neural substrates and cognition have been created on the basis of brain activations, sets of univariate (location-based) measurements of the level of regional brain activity. If these mappings are indeed accurate and specific, it should be possible to decode specific cognitive states on the basis of observed brain activity. The basic idea is simple. In principle, if two mental states result in differences in brain activation for at least some locations in the brain, these mental states can be inferred. In practice, such "brain reading" is difficult to achieve by examining patterns of brain activation in single locations due to the small size of signal differences as well as the inherently distributed character of neural activity. Multivariate pattern-based analyses are significantly more successful as they take advantage of distributed information about mental states carried by activity in multiple locations (Haynes and Rees, 2006). Machine learning and statistical pattern recognition techniques can be employed to achieve optimal separation between different patterns of brain activity and thus to increase detection accuracy. Decoding of mental states has been attempted in the context of visual object recognition, capitalizing on known differences in the pattern of neural responses to different object categories (Haxby et al., 2001). Functional specialization in the visual cortex results in spatial separation of brain activation for images of faces and buildings. These local differences allow observers to accurately track visual perception for at least some object categories. Extending this paradigm to spontaneous changes in visual perception such as those experienced in binocular rivalry, a pattern classifier trained to distinguish fMRI response patterns to the two perceptual alternatives can be used to predict perceptual fluctuations as they occur in real time (Haynes and Rees, 2005).[12]

However, when interpreting relationships between cognition and brain activity, one must be mindful of caveats relating to the "reverse inference" of mental states from brain states. We stated above that once a mapping between mental states and neural responses has been established, it should be possible to infer mental states from neural observations. However, the logic of this argument is flawed—the mapping from mental state to neural response can only be reliably inverted if there is a one-to-one mapping between these two domains, that is, a specific neural response is seen *if and only if* a specific mental state occurs (Poldrack, 2006). That, however, is not the case, given the nature of brain networks and their distributed responses to essentially all exogenous or endogenous perturbations (stimuli and tasks). The degree to which neural responses can provide evidence about mental processes can be quantified since it depends on the degree to which local responses vary across the repertoire of mental or cognitive states. Put differently, the selectivity of a brain region's response in a variety of contexts can provide an estimate of the evidence the region provides about the presence of specific mental states. Russ Poldrack has conducted extensive statistical analyses of large databases reporting on focal brain activations in response to a broad spectrum of cognitive tasks. These studies depend on the ability to access and mine large numbers of fMRI studies. In a recent effort combining automated text mining, meta-analysis, and machine learning approaches, Yarkoni et al. (2011) constructed a database called NeuroSynth that allows both forward and reverse inference (http://neurosynth.org). The framework allows for decoding of a broad range of cognitive and psychological states in individual subjects on the basis of distributed patterns of brain activity and at a high level of accuracy.

Reverse inference or brain reading relies on an accurate classification of mental processes, a cognitive ontology. Text-mining tools and pattern classifiers depend on the prior definition of these categories to establish mind–brain relationships. How can one improve on the relatively coarse cognitive ontology that is currently employed, and can such an ontology be objectively extracted from brain data? Building a map of major concepts and relations for human mental processing is akin to identifying a low-dimensional space that best represents cognitive or psychological states. Each dimension corresponds to a mental category, or a related set of cognitive and behavioral capacities. Poldrack et al. (2009) attempted to map brain activation patterns obtained from a cohort of participants engaged in a variety of cognitive tasks onto a low-dimensional space. These dimensions may be viewed as corresponding to high-dimensional "features" of functional brain activation and contribute to each of the cognitive tasks to a varying degree. A simple ontology of mental processes was successfully mapped onto these dimensions, thus suggesting a correlation between mental architecture and its distributed neural substrate.

An appealing hypothesis is that categories of mental processes are related to distinct brain networks, for example, those identified in studies of the resting-state functional connectome (see chapter 6). As we reviewed earlier, longtime averages of correlations in spontaneous BOLD signal fluctuations allow the identification of several resting-state networks, varying in number depending on scan resolution and clustering technique. Several "canonical networks" primarily involved in default mode, attention, executive control, salience, sensorimotor, visual, and auditory processing are reliably found (Raichle, 2011; see figure 6.6). Using ICA, Smith et al. (2009) identified major components in BOLD time series with significant shared signal variance (i.e., coherent subsystems; see figure 6.8). These components were found to be significantly related to regional activations in various tasks. Thus, functional brain networks can be correlated with distinct cognitive challenges. Displayed in matrix format (figure 8.6), it appears that each distinct cognitive or behavioral domain is associated with a unique pattern of activity engaging a subset of network components. Building on

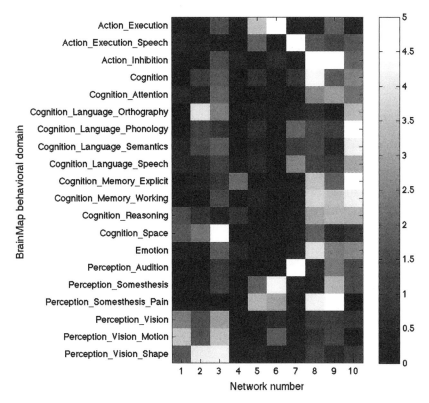

Figure 8.6
Association between brain networks and domains of behavior and cognition. Brain networks are numbered 1 to 10 and correspond to the ICA-derived spatial maps shown in figure 6.8. Behavioral domains are a subset of 66 categories defined in the BrainMap database, which is a large repository of functional magnetic resonance imaging and positron emission tomography brain activation studies (Fox and Lancaster, 2002). The matrix entries express the strength (in arbitrary units) of the association of a given network with a given behavioral domain, as determined by the comparison of each network's spatial signature against activation data in BrainMap. Modified (converted to grayscale) and reproduced with permission from Smith et al., 2009.

the association of cognitive processes and resting-state networks, two studies (Richiardi et al., 2011; Shirer et al., 2012) have successfully used whole-brain functional connectivity to decode mental states occurring in the course of spontaneous cognition, both within and across individuals.

The emerging picture is one where multiple regions and networks are associated with multiple cognitive tasks or mental processes. Building on large-scale databases and automated clustering and machine learning approaches, efforts are under way to extract "functional ontologies" that systematically record which uni- and multivariate brain activation patterns, or functional networks, map onto which domain of cognition.[13] The utility of any functional and/or cognitive ontology depends on its ability to efficiently and accurately translate structure (neural substrate) into function (task or cognitive state) and back (Price and Friston, 2005). The connectome will turn out to be an important ingredient for creating this ontology. The architecture of the human connectome will allow us to anchor cognitive ontology in network connectivity, thus providing a structural foundation for the major categories of human mental processes.

The Next Ten Years

In the near future, computational approaches to connectomics will likely undergo rapid expansion, particularly in the areas of shared neuroinformatics resources, network analysis, and modeling. The increasingly broad availability of high-quality data on human structural and functional connectivity, together with matching data on behavior and genomics, as, for example, planned in the context of the Human Connectome Project, will open new opportunities for both discovery science and hypothesis-driven investigation. The complex relationship between genotype and connectional or behavioral phenotype will be a prime target of analysis, aided by new metrics to extract characteristic patterns of local and global network architecture. These analyses will, for the first time, provide invaluable information on the genetic basis and behavioral manifestations of connectome topology.

A major rationale for mapping the human connectome is to learn more about the role of connectional disturbances in brain dysfunction and disease. Numerous studies have already been conducted, and many more are under way, to probe for differences in the layout of structural and functional connections between healthy and diseased brains. Some of these studies suggest that network theory applied to connectome maps may supply long-sought objective biomarkers for common diseases of the nervous system. Throughout the book, we have underscored the importance of structural connectivity for the specificity of neural responses and for their system-wide integration. Supporting this idea, there is strong evidence suggesting a relationship between specific aspects of network organization and cognitive performance among cohorts of healthy volunteers. The approach is readily extended to include clinical populations. While most studies so far consider disease conditions as categorically different from a healthy state, following a case/control design, new views suggest that disorders represent extreme variations along continuous dimensions and are thus quantitative rather than qualitative deviations from health (Hyman, 2010; Kendler et al., 2011).[14] This idea is concordant with a genetic basis for many common diseases that represents the accumulation of small effects contributed by numerous genetic variants rather than the presence or absence of single genetic factors (Plomin et al., 2009). Thus, common disease conditions, including those affecting the nervous system and resulting in psychopathology, may be best understood as quantitative traits that represent the extremes of otherwise continuous phenotypic distributions. Given the variability of individual brain connectivity (see chapter 3) and its partial heritability, an attractive hypothesis suggests that dimensional variations of connectivity measures can capture neurobiological substrates for multiple forms of brain and mental disorders. Some of these disorders, particularly those that share common genetic bases and show comorbidity, may vary along common dimensions.

Today, "personal genomics" is just over the horizon. "Personal connectomics" may not be far behind. If (as the author anticipates) the connectome turns out to be of clinical importance, and if its status as an important phenotypic maker of individual behavioral and cognitive performance is confirmed, personal connectomes may become integral components of individual medical records. For example, individual connectome maps may be helpful in designing optimal strategies for "network recovery" following traumatic brain injury or stroke (see, e.g., Irimia et al., 2012). People who are at high risk of sustaining such injuries may benefit from the preemptive acquisition of a whole-brain connectome map, to establish a reference or ground state that can guide therapeutic strategies aiming at restoring connectivity in case of brain trauma. Connectome maps may also provide important tools for tracking progressive changes in brain connectivity in individuals with a degenerative brain disease, thus continually providing specific information about the status of the biological substrate and allowing more targeted intervention or therapy.

Genome and connectome are undoubtedly important biological substrates of human individuality. However, this notion, when pushed too far, greatly overstates the deterministic power of genes and connections. While it is certainly true that genome and connectome jointly preserve a record of natural history and personal experience, their translation into biological form and function results from processes and systems that range over many scales of organization. Function emerges from the expression of genes and connections in morphogenesis and development, culminating in complex brain dynamics that underpin the behavior and mental experience of each living individual. The connectome, like the genome, cannot be read like a book. The connectome must express itself in dynamics and behavior before the information it contains can be realized and understood. As the connectome is set in motion, fast and slow fluctuations of neuronal activity give rise to the intrinsic flow of mental experience, molded by the gradual accumulation of structural changes that retain traces of a person's interaction with the physical and social world. The connectome constrains what is possible, but it does not determine what actually occurs. Along the winding path of each person's unique life story, much of what matters most remains irreducible.

Epilogue

This book has covered a wide range of topics, all of them related to the nascent field of connectomics. Let us look back and review some of the main ideas.

• Exemplifying the fundamental role of structure for biological function, the connectome delivers a structural description of the network of connections comprising the human brain. The network architecture of the connectome informs our understanding of the brain as an integrated system, and the empirical and computational strategies of connectomics resemble those of modern systems biology.

• While the primary objective of connectomics is the mapping of structural brain connectivity, knowledge of the structure alone is insufficient for understanding brain function. Neural activity unfolding within the "wiring diagram" of the brain gives rise to complex dynamics characterized by a large repertoire of spatial and temporal patterns.

• Connectomics faces many challenges, including those posed by the multiscale aspect of connectivity, its considerable variability across individuals, and its plasticity across time. Overcoming these challenges requires the deployment of empirical techniques that can reveal connectivity from the micro- to the macroscale and a focus on populations of individuals to systematically assess connectional variability.

• A broad range of empirical techniques aim to deliver detailed connectivity maps of neurons, circuits, and systems. All scales matter for the functioning of the system as a whole, and technology for integrating connectivity data across scales is urgently needed. One essential tool to achieve this integration is the theoretical framework of network science, and the description of the connectome as a network or graph.

• Current work in human connectomics builds on the capacity of noninvasive neuroimaging technology to infer structural connectivity and observe brain dynamics in relation to human behavior. Since anatomical patterns cannot be directly measured in live humans, existing empirical approaches are subject to important limitations. As these limitations are addressed and results are validated, a more consistent picture of the human connectome begins to emerge.

• Brain dynamics, especially when observed over long periods of time, generates characteristic patterns, summarized in the "functional connectome." Structured by the underlying substrate of synaptic connections, detailed study of functional brain connectivity has led to the definition of characteristic brain networks that participate in different aspects of function and that exhibit individual variability and plasticity.

• Functional networks are not rigidly specified but engage in temporal fluctuations on multiple time scales, forming a repertoire of network states that far transcends the connectome's wiring diagram. The dynamics of functional networks and their propensity for modulation by internal state and external input invalidate any simple-minded attempt to reduce brain function to brain wiring.

• The complex architecture of the human connectome can be described as a network or graph, composed of nodes and edges. The network exhibits highly nonrandom organization, with structural modules that are interlinked by hub nodes and arranged into a nested hierarchy. Network topology reflects a trade-off between conserving connection and metabolic cost while at the same time promoting high efficiency of information flow and neural processing.

• Connectomics increasingly depends on cumulative and integrative efforts to bring together data on connectivity, behavior, and genomics. A growing neuroinformatics infrastructure facilitates efforts to create computational models of the human brain. These "virtual brains" are important tools for understanding how brain structure turns into brain function, and they provide new insights into disease states, brain injury, and repair.

Throughout the book I have attempted to lay out a vision of connectomics that embraces the complexity of the brain and remains faithful to its neurobiology. Connectivity was a central theme in this endeavor, and the creation of a comprehensive map of the brain's connections, from synapses to pathways, constitutes the principal challenge of connectomics. And yet, even if such a complete map of the human connectome were at hand, important questions about how this map relates to human behavior and cognition remain to be addressed. The map alone is not the answer—connectomics must include the study of how circuits give rise to variable neural dynamics and how these dynamics underpin brain function. Like genes, connections must be functionally expressed to exert causal efficacy. Brain function arises from the coordinated action of neural elements organized into a complex multiscale system. The network structure of the connectome provides a fundamental constraint for what is functionally possible and probable.

It is my hope and expectation that connectomics, or "network neuroscience," will not only provide deep insights into how the human brain is organized but also allow us to ask new questions about how brain structure gives rise to brain function. These new questions will illuminate how the connections between neural elements enable integrative and emergent neural processes. I think we'll find that the complex architecture of the connectome and its variable dynamics fundamentally resist reductionist explanation. Instead, connectomics offers a complementary perspective, one that is rooted in thinking about networked systems that are complex, yet robust and resilient, and whose dynamics give rise to a seemingly endless variety of expression—constrained, yet running free.

Notes

Chapter 1

1. Individual protein molecules can be conceptualized as networks of interacting chemical domains. Protein structure networks define the interactions of amino acid residues and are useful models for predicting folding probability, the spatial configuration of the protein as a whole, and the position of active centers (Krishnan et al., 2008).

2. The origins of systems biology go back at least to theoreticians like Ludwig von Bertalanffy and Nicolas Rashevsky, who were among the first to link biological processes to general systems theory (von Bertalanffy, 1968) and quantitative models (Rashevsky, 1948).

3. Winkler referred to the genome as the haploid set of all chromosomes, which represents "the material foundation of the species" ("die materielle Grundlage der systematischen Einheit"; Winkler, 1920, p. 165).

4. The corresponding research areas are denoted with the suffix "omics" as in genomics, proteomics, transciptomics, metabolomics, and interactomics.

5. It should be noted that the connectome (and even, to an extent, the genome) is subject to modification during the lifetime of an organism, an issue I will discuss in much more detail in chapter 3. However, at least at the large-scale of regions and pathways, the basic network architecture of the connectome maintains a consistent pattern across time.

6. In the past, systems biology and computational neuroscience have had little interaction (De Schutter, 2008). Both disciplines are concerned with modeling of biological systems, but from different perspectives. Connectomics offers an attractive opportunity to bring the two complementary research agendas closer together.

7. Data-driven or "inductive" approaches to science are sometimes criticized since they don't view scientific progress as deriving primarily from testing specific hypotheses. A good summary of the argument and a defense of data-driven scientific approaches are given by Kell and Oliver (2004). As they point out, "neither Darwin nor Wallace, at the time they started to collect specimens and make observations of the living world in far-flung parts of the globe, sought to test any specific hypothesis. […] It was only when they started to organize their specimens […] that they entered upon the grand synthesis that is the Theory of Evolution by Natural Selection" (Kell and Oliver, 2004, p. 102).

8. Translation by the author. The original formulation, highlighted in the Introduction to Exner's 1894 book, reads: "Ich betrachte es also als meine Aufgabe, die wichtigsten psychischen Erscheinungen auf die Abstufungen von Erregungszuständen der Nerven and Nervencentren, demnach alles, was uns im Bewusstsein als Mannigfaltigkeit erscheint, auf quantitative Verhältnisse und auf die Verschiedenheit der centralen Verbindungen von sonst wesentlich gleichartigen Nerven und Centren zurückzuführen" (Exner, 1894, p. 3).

9. Echoing Granovetter, neuroscience faces a similar challenge of linking small-scale (e.g., neuronal) to large-scale (e.g., systems) processes.

10. The appeal of the small-world phenomenon in social networks was captured in John Guare's evocative play *Six Degrees of Separation*, which I remember seeing at New York's Lincoln Center in the early 1990s.

11. In principle, the detection of network communities is a clustering problem and can thus be addressed with a broad array of clustering and segmentation algorithms. While these techniques can certainly be productively applied to multivariate brain data, the study of network communities with graph analysis offers some unique advantages. For example, module detection directly leads to quantifying the functional roles of nodes and edges within the graph's community structure and, furthermore, allows an assessment of the network's robustness and vulnerability. Complex networks not only offer a rich repertoire of analytic tools but also represent a theoretical framework for brain function.

12. In China, a parallel effort to map the human brain connectome, dubbed the "Brainnetome," is under way (www.brainnetome.org). The CONNECT consortium funded under the European Union's Framework Programme 7 (www.brain-connect.eu) aims at diffusion imaging of the human brain and plans to use noninvasive brain imaging to link the measurement of structural connectivity across multiple scales.

13. In the wake of the announcement of the NIH's Human Connectome Project, the journal editors of *Nature Neuroscience* took the unusual step of publishing an editorial warning of misconceptions and misrepresentations that may result from an uncritical assessment of connectomics and an overstatement of its potential benefits. Drawing a parallel to the Human Genome Project, the article warned that "given the challenges that this field [connectomics] is facing, it seems ill-advised to present connectomics as providing immediate answers for disease when it is clear that this is a long-term goal [...]" (Editorial, 2010, p. 1441).

14. The link between synaptic wiring (the connectome at the microscale) and human individuality is the core thesis developed in Sebastian Seung's recent book entitled *Connectome—How the Brain's Wiring Makes Us Who We Are* (Seung, 2012).

15. The process by which the Human Genome Project became transformed from an unfunded visionary idea to a concerted and focused effort centered around several U.S. federal science agencies, foremost the NIH, is described in detail in Cook-Deegan (1991). The intriguing intellectual history of the project is more fully charted in Cook-Deegan (1994).

16. The impact of genomics is felt far beyond the biological sciences and has begun to transform medical practice as well as creating enormous new economic opportunities. The U.S. government invested an estimated $3.8 billion in the Human Genome Project. According to a 2011 study carried out by the Battelle Memorial Institute, the project has generated $796 billion in economic impact between 1988 and 2010 for a return on investment of 141 to 1 (Battelle, 2011).

Chapter 2

1. Cajal's monumental work built on or paralleled that of many predecessors and contemporaries, including most notably Theodor Schwann, Albrecht von Kölliker, Wilhelm Waldeyer, Joseph von Gerlach, Fridtjof Nansen, and Camillo Golgi.

2. The term "ground truth" generally refers to an objective reality against which remotely sensed observational data are compared. Inferred or predicted features of models based on observational data can then be validated. A classic example is the comparison of satellite or aerial images, acquired from a great distance and with limited resolution, to objects and features that are actually present "on the ground."

3. The anatomist and geneticist Richard Goldschmidt conducted detailed microscopic analyses of the cellular anatomy of the worm *Ascaris* over 100 years ago. In the introduction to his 1908 account of the structure of the worm's nervous system, Goldschmidt clearly articulated the main rationale for the endeavor: "to obtain the necessary anatomical basis for understanding physiological processes it would be highly desirable to know the com-

plete composition of the nervous system of an organism" (Goldschmidt, 1908, p. 74; translation by the author).

4. The map has been continually refined and updated and includes, in its latest edition (Varshney et al., 2011), 280 neurons, 6,393 chemical synapses, 890 electrical junctions, and 1,410 neuromuscular junctions. The network can be downloaded at http://www.wormatlas .org/neuronalwiring.html.

5. The similarity structure of the matrix was subsequently investigated by Malcolm Young (Young, 1992), who also extended the collation of macaque cortical regions and their interconnections to other sensory and motor domains (Young, 1993). First graph analyses of Felleman and Van Essen's connection matrix focused on the clustered and small-world architecture of the connection patterns (Sporns et al., 2000; Hilgetag et al., 2000).

6. Macaque connectivity is cataloged in the CoCoMac database (www.cocomac.org), originated by Rolf Kötter (Kötter, 2004). Rat connectivity is cataloged in the Brain Architecture Management System (http://brancusi.usc.edu/bkms), curated by Mihail Bota (Bota et al., 2005; Bota and Swanson, 2010). The neuronal structure of the nervous system of *C. elegans* is available at http://www.wormatlas.org/neuronalwiring.html.

7. For a personal perspective on the history of graph theory and the connectome, see Sporns (2012).

8. See http://hebb.mit.edu/courses/connectomics/index07.html.

9. Connection length is particularly important as it is, together with the axonal diameter, a major determinant of the conduction delay and hence of the speed with which information is transmitted. Time delays are critical for system dynamics. Following a suggestion by Viktor Jirsa (Jirsa, 2004), the connectome might be viewed as having a "space–time structure" defining not only which nodes are connected but also the relative timing of impulses sent between them.

10. The connectivity patterns revealed by longtime averages of resting-state functional networks measured by fMRI represent an important exception and form the basis of "functional connectomics" (see chapter 6). These patterns are quite stable within and across individuals and provide important information about functional brain systems. It is likely that they derive much of their consistency from the underlying anatomy of structural pathways (see chapter 6).

11. In the run-up to the completion of the human genome sequence, estimates for the number of genes ranged rather widely, from less than 30,000 to more than 150,000 (Pennisi, 2000). We now know that the number is far lower than most experts had originally predicted, perhaps less than 25,000 and thus only slightly greater than the number of genes in *C. elegans*. It is worth noting that despite the fact that sequences have now been available for over a decade, the exact number of genes comprising the human genome is still unknown, due to the difficulty of segmenting coding from noncoding regions (a problem of genomic parcellation, analogous to connectomic parcellation; see chapter 5).

12. Data on the number, sizes, and interconnections of cortical regions of various mammalian species suggest robust scaling relationships relative to brain volume. Extrapolating from these data to the human brain, Changizi and Shimojo (2005) projected that human neocortex contains approximately 150 brain areas, with on average 60 connections per area, for a total of 9,000 distinct interareal connections. David Van Essen has independently estimated a total of 100 to 200 anatomically distinct areas for human cortex (Van Essen, 2004). Using a combination of task-evoked and spontaneous neural activity measured with fMRI, Power et al. (2011) devised a parcellation scheme that resulted in 264 cortical and subcortical regions within one brain hemisphere.

13. Dense connectome mapping may be contrasted with sparse mapping strategies that require overlay and assembly of structural information sampled from multiple individuals.

14. The idea that neuronal circuits could be understood on the basis of statistical properties of ensembles has a long history. McCulloch and Pitts wrote in 1948 that "the nervous system

as a whole is ordered and operated on statistical principles" (McCulloch and Pitts, 1948, p. 98), and the neuroanatomist D. A. Sholl argued in 1956 for a statistical description of neural circuits: "Histological studies show that no theory [...] relying on specific circuits can be maintained. The alternative approach must depend upon statistical considerations in which the connections of individual neurons are of less concern and the connectivity pattern of the neuronal aggregates is studied" (Sholl, 1956, p. 102).

15. Two copies of human DNA, the molecules measuring about 4 meters in length, are densely packed and folded into each cell's nucleus. The locations of chromosomes and individual genes within the nucleus are highly nonrandom and linked to transcriptional activity and coordinate gene expression. It is unclear to what extent these spatially defined functional interactions depend on long-range correlations present in coding and noncoding DNA sequences (e.g., Audit et al., 2001).

16. "Whether it be the sweeping eagle in his flight or the open apple blossom, the toiling work horse, the blithe swan, the branching oak, the winding stream at its base, the drifting clouds, over all the coursing sun, form ever follows function" (Sullivan, 1896, p. 403).

17. The problem and its history are lucidly presented in Schall (2004).

Chapter 3

1. In contrast, establishing the anatomical and functional correspondence of individual neurons across individuals is often possible (to a degree) in invertebrate species.

2. Paul Nunez refers to the (in his view undeserved and unjustified) emphasis on a single scale for understanding brain function as "scale chauvinism" (e.g., Nunez, 2000).

3. The estimate is based on binary representations of mammalian cortex derived from tract-tracing studies over several decades (see chapter 5). More recent reexamination of interregional pathways in mammalian cortex with quantitative tracer methods suggests that a majority of areas are directly connected and that the connection density varies over up to five orders of magnitude (e.g., Markov et al., 2011).

4. It also poses a major theoretical problem for relating psychological and cognitive function to neural substrates. Aizawa and Gillett (2009) discuss the problem in the context of the "massive multiple realization hypothesis," which states that human psychological (cognitive, behavioral) properties are found to be associated with a great number of multiple realizations of properties and mechanisms at different levels of neurobiology. This notion, if indeed correct, may be viewed as supporting the idea that the study of cognition is autonomous with respect to neuroscience since neuroscience cannot deliver a unique set of neurobiological elements and properties that are required for human cognition to emerge. In the present context of connectomics, an attractive hypothesis suggests that what matters most for human cognition are specific aspects of network organization that are invariant across multiple realizations (see chapter 7).

5. It appears that the individual variability of the volume of the primary visual cortex is greater than the variability of cortical volume as a whole (Glissen and Zilles, 1995).

6. A recent systematic study of molecular turnover in mouse fibroblasts examined the dynamics of more than 5,000 different mRNA and proteins (Schwanhäusser et al., 2011). Proteins were found to have a median half-life of 46 hours, with only a very small percentage reaching half-lives longer than 200 hours. Proteins with greater stability were mainly involved in "housekeeping" processes such as cellular respiration, ribosomal translation, glycolysis, and the citric acid cycle.

7. Some studies have examined the development of structural connectivity in nonhuman mammalian species. For example, diffusion spectrum imaging has been used to map cortical tracts at various developmental stages in the cat brain (Takahashi et al., 2010).

8. Genetic terminology is deeply imbued with metaphors that refer to the genome as "information," which is "encoding" phenotypes and is "translated" or "read-out" during protein synthesis. Among the general public, this notion of "genome-as-text," comprising the "book of life," is widespread, reflected, for example, in public statements of political

leaders. In their joint press conference on June 26, 2000, announcing the completion of the first DNA sequence of the human genome, U.S. President Bill Clinton remarked that "today, we are learning the language in which God created life" while British Prime Minister Tony Blair called it "a working blueprint of the human race." Such rhetoric vastly underestimates the complex relationship between the genetic material and its instantiation in biological form and function.

9. Sequencing of the first human genome came at the cost of several hundred million U.S. dollars and took many months of work. Since then, the cost of whole genome sequencing has fallen dramatically, to less than $100,000 in 2008, and around $5,000 in 2009. In January 2012, the biotech company Life Technologies announced a new device designed to sequence a human genome in a day, for a cost of less than $1,000. Ultimately that price tag may decrease to as little as $100. None of these estimates figure in the considerable cost involved in making sense of these data.

Chapter 4

1. Dendritic branches add a further 500 meters to the wiring diagram, according to Braitenberg and Schüz (1998), who arrived at these estimates based on an analysis of mouse cortex. Data on human brain indicate that a total length of around 220 meters of axonal length is contained in each cubic millimeter of cerebral white matter, which given a white matter volume of approximately 500–700 cm^3 adds to between 110,000 and 150,000 km of aggregate axonal length (Pakkenberg et al., 2003).

2. The earth's land surface extends over approximately 150 million km^2. Imaging at 1 m^2 resolution (a common resolution found in Google Earth 6.0) with 8 bits per voxel results in 1.5×10^{14} bytes (0.15 petabyte) of data. Thus, a high-resolution map of the entire earth corresponds to one tenth of the data coming from EM microscopy of 1 mm^3 of neural tissue.

3. Informal estimates indicate that mapping only 1 mm^3 of neural tissue would take thousands of work years with current technology. Helmstaedter et al. (2011) suggested that the full contouring of every neurite in a $100 \times 100 \times 100$ μm^3 volume would consume 60,000 hours of work and that following individual neurites in EM volumes would require a decision about continuing, terminating, or branching (leaving aside spines and synapses) roughly every 4 μm, resulting in a total of 100 million decisions for a single mouse cortical column containing 400 meters of neurites.

4. To stimulate progress in this area, a competition called DIADEM challenge (DIgital reconstructions of Axonal and DEndridic Morphology) was held in 2009–2010. Registered teams participated by developing automated neuronal reconstruction algorithms that were scored on specific data sets. New approaches to automated reconstruction are viewed as a "neuroinformatics grand challenge," an essential milestone toward comprehensive circuit mapping (Ascoli, 2008).

5. Hama et al. (2011) recently introduced a very different approach to imaging brain connectivity, relying on fluorescent labeling of anatomical structures combined with a technique to render the brain volume translucent. Using this approach, the authors were able to image and trace deep regions and pathways of the mouse brain.

6. A related strategy for reconstructing synaptic connectivity with the aid of fluorescent markers has been suggested by Mishchenko (2011).

7. As Stephen J. Smith has suggested, the complete set of structurally and functionally distinct synapses might be called the "synaptome." In a slightly different sense, the term has also been proposed by De Felipe (2010).

8. The enteric division of the autonomic nervous system consists of approximately 100 million neurons that are embedded in the wall of the gastrointestinal tract. The operation of this system is vital to ensure proper functioning of the digestive system. Capable of autonomous operation, the enteric division contains more motor neurons than the entire spinal cord as well as a large percentage of the body's neuromodulators. Its connectome is

entirely unmapped. I am not aware of anyone who has stepped forward to take on this sobering assignment.

Chapter 5

1. Meynert discovered numerous important neuroanatomical structures including the nucleus basalis and the habenular-peduncular tract.

2. In addition to efforts under way in the mouse brain, data on rat brain connectivity have also been rendered into a connectome (network) format. An interactive database on rat hippocampal and retrosplenial connections has recently been compiled by Sugar et al. (2011), and a complete map of the connections among cell types of the hippocampus (the "hippocampome") is on the horizon (Ascoli, 2010).

3. The inferential nature of structural connectivity data obtained from diffusion imaging sets it apart from other more direct ways of observing anatomical connections—for example, with classical anatomy or microscopy. However, while these more classical techniques are often designated as the "ground truth," they still face difficult obstacles when attempting precise quantification of anatomical relationships and the uniform assessment of connectivity across a whole brain. Statistical approaches necessarily enter into descriptions of connectivity even when more direct anatomical measures are pursued.

4. This approach is particularly appropriate for random or atlas-based parcellations. In more objective parcellations that identify functionally coherent brain regions, the uncorrected streamline count might be more appropriate. Further corrections for various biases introduced by imaging or tractography can be applied. For example, in deterministic streamline tractography connection densities may be normalized by fiber length since longer connections traverse greater numbers of voxels and are therefore more likely to be seeded in the initial reconstruction step (Hagmann et al., 2007, 2008).

5. Significant inroads have also been made in other "model organisms" such as the mouse, where noninvasive imaging of anatomical connectivity is now possible (Jiang and Johnson, 2011). Rodent anatomy also provides an excellent test bed for validation of noninvasive diffusion imaging approaches (e.g., Leergaard et al., 2010), and a recently compiled population-averaged DTI atlas for the rat brain may be useful for relating diffusion imaging to tract tracing data (Veraart et al., 2011).

6. For a historical perspective on the classical cytoarchitectonic map described by Korbinian Brodmann in 1909, see Zilles and Amunts (2010).

7. To drive home this point, imagine randomly partitioning the earth into patches of land while attempting to chart social or economic interactions. A randomly partitioned map of Europe would, for example, greatly diminish the distinctive contributions of nations or geographic communities at a scale below the average parcel size (for an instructive figure, see Wig et al., 2011). Instead, partitioning geography based on patterns of human transactions (human "functional connectivity") provides a much better way to reveal cohesive social and economic regions (e.g., Ratti et al., 2010).

8. The idea that connectivity defines function was perhaps most clearly expressed by Marcel Mesulam: "Nothing defines the function of a neuron more faithfully than the nature of its inputs and outputs" (Mesulam, 2005, p. 6).

9. Eickhoff et al. (2011) have argued that cortical modules or parcels derived on the basis of structural and/or functional connectivity have to be aligned with information from task-evoked activations. In their approach, comprehensive data on brain activations across task is combined through "meta-analytic connectivity mapping" to yield information on patterns of functional segregation.

Chapter 6

1. Networks of interacting molecules can be viewed as processing information (Missiuro et al., 2009), and the centrality of proteins in cellular information flow is predictive of its importance for global network integrity.

2. The term "functional connectivity" refers to an estimate of the statistical dependence between spatially separated neurophysiological time series, often expressed as a simple cross-correlation. This is a "functional" estimate only insofar as it is obtained from a functioning brain—functional connectivity generally does not imply a causative role of the measured dependencies in a specific functional process.

3. Functional connectivity can be measured even between neural elements in the brains of different people that are engaged in social interaction (Anders et al., 2011) or viewing a common source of input—for example, a movie (Hasson et al., 2004). Clearly, the source of the statistical dependence in these cases is found in the environment; it is not due to causal effects mediated by the anatomy. It is also important to remember that long-range correlations can also arise as a result of global coherence in a system of locally coupled elements, for example, a spin glass.

4. Callosotomy does not always involve cutting all interhemispheric communication paths. Fibers traveling in the anterior commissure may be spared, and indirect synaptic paths through the thalamus are unperturbed.

5. In contrast with these results obtained acutely after callosotomy, two recent studies of persons with agenesis of the corpus callosum revealed significant interhemisperic functional connectivity at rest (Khanna et al., 2011; Tyszka et al., 2011). These functional connections likely result from subcortical structural pathways that compensate for the lack of direct corticocortical structural connections.

6. A comprehensive analysis of a range of methods for extracting functional and effective connections from fMRI data sets (Smith et al., 2011) concluded that covariance-based methods perform reasonably well while lag-based methods such as Granger causality perform relatively poorly. The study also once again demonstrated the importance of accurate parcellation for deriving sound estimates of interregional relationships.

7. BOLD fluctuations and the resulting functional connectivity can also be measured in animal models, for example, nonhuman primates (Vincent et al., 2007; Hutchison et al., 2011; Adachi et al., 2011; Mantini et al., 2011), as well as in rat (Pawela et al., 2008) and mouse (White et al., 2011).

8. The brain accounts for only about 2 percent of total body mass but consumes approximately 20 percent of all energy (Clarke and Sokoloff, 1999). Of that amount, roughly 80 percent is devoted to neuronal signaling processes, including action potentials and post-synaptic potentials (Attwell and Laughlin, 2001)—the estimated "signaling-related energy use of 30 μmol ATP/g/min is equal to that in human leg muscle running the marathon" (Attwell and Laughlin, 2001, p. 1143).

9. The relation between the location of the default mode network, regionally elevated aerobic glycolysis, and distributions of β-amyloid, a key molecule involved in degenerative brain disease, has been noted in several studies (Vlassenko et al., 2010; Drzezga et al. 2011).

10. The link between the level of regional brain metabolism and connection patterns was further explored in recent work on correlations between gray matter structure and connectivity (Varkuti et al., 2011).

11. Lehmann has referred to these microstates as basic building blocks of mental experience, the "atoms of thought" (Lehmann, 1990).

12. The temporal dynamics of interactions within and among resting-state networks as recorded with fMRI are best visualized in movie format. A movie of windowed cross-correlations sampled over a 30-minute period can be downloaded from ftp://imaging.wustl.edu/pub/raichlab/restless_brain/movies/correlation/ (Raichle, 2011). The longtime average of these correlations can be seen in figure 6.6.

13. A stronger version of the idea postulates that genetic or environmental factors that have no impact on the connectome also do not contribute to disease processes. Put yet another way, if connectivity is the final common path to brain and mental disease, then the causal role of genetic or environmental perturbations in pathogenesis should be directly correlated with their deleterious effects on brain networks.

Chapter 7

1. A small number of studies have been carried out using cross-correlations in gray matter volume or thickness across populations of subjects (see chapter 5). However, the biological basis for the relationship between these correlations and the presence of structural connections remains unclear, and the approach may not distinguish between direct and indirect structural pathways.

2. The robustness of graph measures under varying parcellations (Zalesky et al., 2010b) and in test–retest conditions (Wang et al., 2011a) is an important topic of methodological investigation. It should be noted that graph measures can only report robust and reproducible results if sound data acquisition and preprocessing strategies are employed. Noisy imaging, registration errors, faulty parcellation, or excessively short resting-state fMRI runs will introduce undesired variability, and graph measures cannot give consistent results under those circumstances.

3. At present it is unclear how these differences in the number and diversity of projections across cortical regions relate to regional differences in neuron densities (Collins et al., 2010). Contrary to earlier data suggesting structural uniformity across cortex (Rockel et al., 1980), Collins and colleagues reported that neuron densities vary several-fold between cortical regions of the macaque. Primary sensory regions such as V1 have the highest cell densities. However, neither tract tracing nor diffusion tractography confer highest degree or projection density to V1 or other primary sensory cortical areas.

4. It is by no means obvious that all neuronal communication should follow along the shortest paths only. As neurons emit signals or "messages" these signals may propagate along many different alternative routes, as it is not clear that such messages carry "address labels" that specify their intended targets as well as routing instructions. An alternative model to targeted routing of messages is provided by random walks or diffusion (e.g., Costa and Travieso, 2007; Costa et al., 2007).

5. The notion of hierarchy is used here as a way of describing a topologically nested network architecture that can be decomposed into modules at different scales. This mode of network organization does not imply centralized control or serial processing as more common notions of hierarchy in control systems. The contrast between network and hierarchical models of brain architecture is discussed further in Thompson and Swanson (2010).

6. Positive assortativity is more pronounced in structural brain networks that are parcellated into a large number of regions—for example, in random parcellations that divide the brain into hundreds or thousands of nodes. This is an example of how graph metrics can depend on node definition (see chapter 5). Interestingly, the only example so far of a cellular connectome, coming from the invertebrate nervous system of *C. elegans*, exhibits negative assortativity. It remains to be seen if different patterns of assortativity are indicative of fundamental differences in brain topology at large versus small scales or in vertebrates versus invertebrates.

7. Interhemispheric connections, particularly among cortical regions that are farther away from the midline, continue to be difficult to detect with diffusion imaging and tractography. It is possible that the prominence of callosal projections along the medial wall is due to methodological bias. Alternatively, a gradient of interhemispheric connection density away from the midline would be consistent with wiring conservation.

8. Think of the central location of the hub of a bicycle or ferris wheel, or of the orbital hubs in Iain Banks's Culture universe.

9. Dubai's emergence as a global air transportation hub is partly attributed to an explicit hub-and-spoke strategy espoused by major airlines like Etihad and Emirates.

10. Numerous early studies of connectivity have explored the spatiality of brain networks. For example, the relationship between spatial distance and topological connectivity was explored in work by Malcolm Young (Young, 1992), and the role of allometric scaling in shaping connectivity over evolutionary time was recognized long ago by Chuck Stevens, James Ringo, and Terry Deacon (Stevens, 1989; Deacon, 1990; Ringo, 1991).

11. One of the clearest and earliest expressions of the idea can be found in the writings of Santiago Ramón y Cajal, who noted in 1899 that "all of the various conformations of the neuron and its various components are simply morphological adaptations governed by laws of conservation for time, space and material" (Cajal, 1995, pp. 115–116).

12. The idea that connectivity-driven tensile forces influence cortical folding was first proposed by David Van Essen (Van Essen, 1997; see also Herculano-Houzel et al., 2010).

13. Computation and dynamics are sometimes seen as opposite rather than related forces. I once heard Melanie Mitchell cogently expressing their relation in a lecture by defining computation as "dynamics with a purpose."

14. In the end, the human brain may not be as special as it is sometimes made out to be. It is neither the largest, nor, possibly, the most complex nervous system in the known universe. The brain of an adult elephant is about four times the weight of a human brain and contains two to three times more neurons (Williams and Herrup, 1988).

15. For example, this could be accomplished by imaging and tractography, followed by network analysis, of preserved brains of a number of species (Wedeen et al., 2009, 2012).

Chapter 8

1. Remarkably, that number is close to the 30 million dollars allocated by the NIH for the Human Connectome Project at its inception in 2010. The cost of mapping the human brain at the ultrastructural level, however, would still far exceed the amount predicted by Merkle 20 years ago.

2. For the year 2007, the world's data storage capacity, including all media from electronic storage to books and newspapers, was estimated at 295 billion gigabytes (Hilbert and López, 2011) and was thus insufficient to store the complete data of even a single human brain at subcellular resolution. In comparison, storing a single human genome only requires a few gigabytes.

3. These tool sets include the Brain Connectivity Toolbox (Rubinov and Sporns, 2010; www.brain-connectivity-toolbox.net), NetworkX (http://networkx.lanl.gov), NetworkWork-Bench (http://nwb.cns.iu.edu), Pajek (http://pajek.imfm.si), and the visualization package Circos (http://circos.ca).

4. Numerous open-access databases have been created to facilitate progress and collaboration in genomics, for example, a gene-expression atlas of the mouse developing and adult central nervous system (GENSAT; http://www.gensat.org).

5. One of these initiatives, the Open Connectome Project (http://openconnectomeproject.org/) explicitly encourages data sharing across connectome methodologies, from EM to MRI.

6. The project was the first to make large numbers of resting-state fMRI data sets freely available to the scientific community. Among its principal goals is to enable the study of variability in brain–behavior relations. This goal parallels that of the 1000 Genomes Project (http://www.1000genomes.org), an international public–private consortium that was launched in 2008 and aims to collect genomic data from about 2,500 people in 27 populations around the world. Pilot data sets are already freely available to biomedical researchers.

7. The Allen Institute for Brain Science is currently compiling a multimodal atlas for gene expression in the human brain, including genomic data from microarray and in situ hybridization studies as well as anatomical data from MR imaging, building on an earlier effort in mouse brain (Dong, 2007; Lein et al., 2007).

8. Similar ideas have been articulated by Duncan Watts (Watts, 2007). An extremely ambitious proposal to create a "Living Earth Simulator" was put forward by Dirk Helbing and colleagues, as part of a 10-year, 1 billion Euro project that would be funded by the European Commission (http://www.futurict.ethz.ch). The model would allow detailed simulation and forecasting of social, technological, and environmental systems on a planetary scale.

9. More recently, the same group of researchers conducted a simulation of 1.6 billion neurons connected by 9 trillion synapses. The model was run on one of the fastest super-computers in the world, which consumed 1 megawatt of electrical power and occupied an acre-sized room filled with over 147,000 processors and many miles of wiring.

10. In August 2011, researchers at IBM led by Dharmendra Modha were awarded $21 million by the U.S. Defense Advanced Research Projects Agency to develop a new genera-tion of neurosynaptic chips that allow the implementation of neural architectures in computing hardware (http://www-03.ibm.com/press/us/en/pressrelease/35251.wss). Working prototypes contain 256 neurons and thousands of programmable or learning synapses. Eventual applications might include the simulation of an entire connectome at synaptic resolution (Modha et al., 2011).

11. Some advocates of "whole brain emulation" have proposed that a detailed simulation of a functioning artificial human brain can be achieved within a matter of years. The futurist Ray Kurzweil has calculated that with 100 trillion connections performing 200 calculations per second the human brain carries out 20 million billion calculations per second. Given current trends in hardware development computing machinery, matching this performance should be available by the year 2020 (Kurzweil, 2000). Others have, rather optimistically, suggested that brain simulations will enable "mind downloading" and thus allow humans to achieve cognitive immortality (Sandberg and Bostrom, 2008).

12. Brain reading has many potential applications. For example, the accurate decoding of brain signals is an important component of prosthetic devices that operate on the basis of user-generated neural activity. Other applications are considerably more controversial, ranging from using data on mental responses in marketing and advertising to "deception detection." Despite current limitations in the range and accuracy of brain reading, concerns have been raised about the protection of "mental privacy" against involuntary or intrusive practices.

13. Poldrack et al. (2011; see also Yarkoni et al., 2010) have recently launched an effort to create a cumulative knowledge base (ontology) for cognitive neuroscience called the Cog-nitive Atlas (http://www.cognitiveatlas.org). The goal is to provide a systematic description of human mental processes and the tasks that are used to manipulate these processes in cognitive experiments.

14. The problem of diagnosing mental disorders on the basis of categorical distinctions has led to intensive discussions among clinicians and basic scientists in the run-up to the release of the new edition of the *Diagnostic and Statistical Manual of Mental Disorders* (fifth edition) by the American Psychiatric Association, planned for May 2013. Critics point to the relative lack of objective diagnostic criteria based on genetics or neuroimaging and question the emphasis on cataloguing individual disorders rather than representing them as dimensional phenomena with shared symptoms, possibly driven by shared endopheno-types. In the future, connectome analysis may contribute important new objective metrics and can help to define meaningful dimensions of variation and relations between disorders (e.g., Insel et al., 2010).

References

Adachi Y, Osada T, Sporns O, Watanabe T, Matsui T, et al. 2012. Functional connectivity between anatomically unconnected areas is shaped by collective network-level effects in the macaque cortex. *Cereb Cortex* doi: 10.1093/cercor/bhr234.

Aertsen AM, Gerstein GL, Habib MK, Palm G. 1989. Dynamics of neuronal firing correlation: Modulation of "effective connectivity." *J Neurophysiol* 61: 900–917.

Aitchison JD, Galitski T. 2003. Inventories to insights. *J Cell Biol* 161: 465–469.

Aizawa K, Gillett C. 2009. Levels, individual variation, and massive multiple realization in neurobiology. In: Bickle J (ed.), *The Oxford Handbook of Philosophy and Neuroscience*, pp. 539–581. New York: Oxford University Press.

Akil H, Martone ME, Van Essen DC. 2011. Challenges and opportunities in mining neuroscience data. *Science* 331: 708–712.

Alexander DC, Hubbard PL, Hall MG, Moore EA, Ptito M, et al. 2010. Orientationally invariant indices of axon diameter and density from diffusion MRI. *Neuroimage* 52: 1374–1389.

Alstott J, Breakspear M, Hagmann P, Cammoun L, Sporns O. 2009. Modeling the impact of lesions in the human brain. *PLoS Comput Biol* 5: e1000408.

Ananthanarayanan R, Esser SK, Simon HD, Modha DS. 2009. The cat is out of the bag: Cortical simulations with 109 neurons and 1013 synapses. In: Proceedings of the conference on high performance computing networking, storage and analysis, pp. 1–12, New York: ACM.

Anders S, Heinzle J, Weiskopf N, Ethofer T, Haynes JD. 2011. Flow of affective information between communicating brains. *Neuroimage* 54: 439–446.

Anderson JR, Jones BW, Watt CB, Shaw MV, Yang JH, et al. 2011. Exploring the retinal connectome. *Mol Vis* 17: 355–379.

Andrews TJ, Halpern SD, Purves D. 1997. Correlated size variations in human visual cortex, lateral geniculate nucleus, and optic tract. *J Neurosci* 17: 2859–2868.

Anwander A, Tittgemeyer M, von Cramon DY, Friederici AD, Knösche TR. 2007. Connectivity-based parcellation of Broca's area. *Cereb Cortex* 17: 816–825.

Ascoli GA. 2008. Neuroinformatics grand challenges. *Neuroinformatics* 6: 1–3.

Ascoli G. 2010. The coming of age of the hippocampome. *Neuroinformatics* 8: 1–3.

Ashburner M, Ball CA, Blake JA, Botstein D, Butler H, et al. 2000. Gene ontology: Tool for the unification of biology. The Gene Ontology Consortium. *Nat Genet* 25: 25–29.

Attwell D, Laughlin SB. 2001. An energy budget for signaling in the grey matter of the brain. *J Cereb Blood Flow Metab* 21: 1133–1145.

Audit B, Thermes C, Vaillant C, d'Aubenton-Carafa Y, Muzy JF, et al. 2001. Long-range correlations in genomic DNA: A signature of the nucleosomal structure. *Phys Rev Lett* 86: 2471–2474.

Axer M, Amunts K, Graessel D, Palm C, Dammers J, et al. 2011. A novel approach to the human connectome: Ultra-high resolution mapping of fibre tracts in the brain. *Neuroimage* 54: 1091–1101.

Barabási AL, Oltvai ZN. 2004. Network biology: Understanding the cell's functional organization. *Nat Rev Genet* 5: 101–111.

Bard JB, Rhee SY. 2004. Ontologies in biology: Design, applications and future challenges. *Nat Rev Genet* 5: 213–222.

Barrat A, Barthélemy M, Vespignani A. 2005. The effects of spatial constraints on the evolution of weighted complex networks. *J Stat Mech* P05003.

Barthelemy M. 2011. Spatial networks. *Phys Rep* 499: 1–101.

Bascompte J. 2007. Networks in ecology. *Basic Appl Ecol* 8: 485–490.

Basser PJ, Mattiello J, Le Bihan D. 1994. MR diffusion tensor spectroscopy and imaging. *Biophys J* 66: 259–267.

Bassett DS, Bullmore ET. 2006. Small world brain networks. *Neuroscientist* 12: 512–523.

Bassett DS, Bullmore ET, Verchinksi BA, Mattay VS, Weinberger DR, et al. 2008. Hierarchical organization of human cortical networks in health and schizophrenia. *J Neurosci* 28: 9239–9248.

Bassett DS, Bullmore ET. 2009. Human brain networks in health and disease. *Curr Opin Neurol* 22: 340–347.

Bassett DS, Bullmore ET, Meyer-Lindenberg A, Apud JA, Weinberger DR, Coppola R. 2009. Cognitive fitness of cost-efficient brain functional networks. *Proc Natl Acad Sci USA* 106: 11747–11752.

Bassett DS, Greenfield DL, Meyer-Lindenberg A, Weinberger DR, Moore SW, et al. 2010a. Efficient physical embedding of topologically complex information processing networks in brains and computer circuits. *PLoS Comput Biol* 6: e1000748.

Bassett DS, Brown JA, Deshpande V, Carlson JM, Grafton ST. 2010b. Conserved and variable architecture of human white matter connectivity. *Neuroimage* 54: 1262–1279.

Bassett DS, Gazzaniga MS. 2011. Understanding complexity in the human brain. *Trends Cogn Sci* 15: 200–209.

Bassett DS, Wymbs NF, Porter MA, Mucha PJ, Carlson JM, et al. 2011. Dynamic reconfiguration of human brain networks during learning. *Proc Natl Acad Sci USA* 108: 7641–7646.

Battelle. 2011. Economic Impact of the Human Genome Project. A report prepared by Battelle Technology Partnership Practice, May 2011.

Beckmann M, Johansen-Berg H, Rushworth MFS. 2009. Connectivity-based parcellation of human cingulate cortex and its relation to functional specialization. *J Neurosci* 29: 1175–1190.

Beggs JM. 2008. The criticality hypothesis: How local cortical networks might optimize information processing. *Phil Trans R Soc A* 366: 329–343.

Behrens TEJ, Woolrich MW, Jenkinson M, Johansen-Berg H, Nunes RG, et al. 2003. Characterization and propagation of uncertainty in diffusion-weighted MR imaging. *Magn Reson Med* 50: 1077–1088.

Behrens TEJ, Johansen-Berg H, Jbabdi S, Rushworth MFS, Woolrich MW. 2007. Probabilistic diffusion tractography with multiple fibre orientations: What can we gain? *Neuroimage* 34: 144–155.

Behrens TEJ, Sporns O. 2012. Human connectomics. *Curr Opin Neurobiol* 22: 144–153.

Bernhardt BC, Chen Z, He Y, Evans AC, Bernasconi N. 2011. Graph-theoretical analysis reveals disrupted small-world organization of cortical thickness correlation networks in temporal lobe epilepsy. *Cereb Cortex* 21: 2147–2157.

Binzegger T, Douglas RJ, Martin KAC. 2004. A quantitative map of the circuit of cat primary visual cortex. *J Neurosci* 24: 8441–8453.

Binzegger T, Douglas RJ, Martin KAC. 2009. Topology and dynamics of the canonical circuit of cat V1. *Neural Netw* 22: 1071–1078.

Binzegger T, Douglas RJ, Martin KAC. 2010. An axonal perspective on cortical circuits. In: Feldmayer D, Lübke JHR (eds.), *New Aspects of Axonal Structure and Function*, pp. 117–139. Berlin: Springer.

Biswal BB, Mennes M, Zuo XN, Gohel S, Kelly C, et al. 2010. Toward discovery science of human brain function. *Proc Natl Acad Sci USA* 107: 4734–4739.

Bock DD, Lee WCA, Kerlin AM, Andermann ML, Hood G, et al. 2011. Network anatomy and in vivo physiology of visual cortical neurons. *Nature* 471: 177–182.

Bohland JW, Wu C, Barbas H, Bokil H, Bota M, et al. 2009. A proposal for a coordinated effort for the determination of brainwide neuroanatomical connectivity in model organisms at a mesoscopic scale. *PLoS Comput Biol* 5: e1000334.

Bohland JW, Bokil H, Pathak SD, Lee CK, Ng L, et al. 2010. Clustering of spatial gene expression patterns in the mouse brain and comparison with classical neuroanatomy. *Methods* 50: 105–112.

Boly M, Phillips C, Tshibanda L, Vanhaudenhuyse A, Schabus M, et al. 2008. Intrinsic brain activity in altered states of consciousness: How conscious is the default mode of brain function? *Ann N Y Acad Sci* 1129: 119–129.

Bonacich P. 1972. Factoring and weighting approaches to clique identification. *J Math Sociol* 2: 113–120.

Bonifazi P, Goldin M, Picardo MA, Jorquera I, Cattani A, et al. 2009. GABAergic hub neurons orchestrate synchrony in developing hippocampal networks. *Science* 326: 1419–1424.

Bota M, Dong HW, Swanson LW. 2005. Brain architecture management system. *Neuroinformatics* 3: 15–48.

Bota M, Swanson LW. 2010. Collating and curating neuroanatomical nomenclatures: Principles and use of the Brain Architecture Knowledge Management System (BAMS). *Front Neuroinf* 4: 3.

Botteron K, Dierker D, Todd R, Alexopolous J, Seung D, et al. 2008. Human vs. computer algorithm choices in identifying identical twin pairs based on cortical shape characteristics: Who's better? Org. Human Brain Mapping Annual Meeting, Abstract #1595.

Boyden ES, Zhang F, Bamberg E, Nagel G, Deisseroth K. 2005. Millisecond-timescale, genetically targeted optical control of neural activity. *Nat Neurosci* 8: 1263–1268.

Braitenberg V. 1990. Reading the structure of brains. *Network* 1: 1–11.

Braitenberg V, Schüz A. 1998. *Statistics and Geometry of Neuronal Connectivity*. Berlin: Springer.

Branco T, Häusser M. 2010. The single dendritic branch as a fundamental functional unit in the nervous system. *Trends Neurosci* 20: 494–502.

Branco T, Clark BA, Häusser M. 2011. Dendritic discrimination of temporal input sequences in cortical neurons. *Science* 329: 1671–1675.

Breakspear M, McIntosh AR. 2011. Networks, noise and models: Reconceptualizing the brain as a complex, distributed system. *Neuroimage* 58: 293–295.

Brezina V. 2010. Beyond the wiring diagram: Signalling through complex neuromodulator networks. *Phil Trans Roy Soc B* 365: 2363–2374.

Briggman KL, Denk W. 2006. Towards neural circuit reconstruction with volume electron microscopy techniques. *Curr Opin Neurobiol* 16: 562–570.

Briggman KL, Bock DD. 2012. Volume electron microscopy for neuronal circuit reconstruction. *Curr Opin Neurobiol* 22: 154–161.

Briggman KL, Helmstaedter M, Denk W. 2011. Wiring specificity in the direction-selectivity circuit of the retina. *Nature* 471: 183–188.

Britz J, Van de Ville D, Michel CM. 2010. BOLD correlates of EEG topography reveal rapid resting-state network dynamics. *Neuroimage* 52: 1162–1170.

Bucher D. 2009. Neuronal homeostasis: Does form follow function or vice versa? *Curr Biol* 19: R64–R67.

Buckner RL, Andrews-Hanna JR, Schacter DL. 2008. The brain's default network: Anatomy, function, and relevance to disease. *Ann N Y Acad Sci* 1124: 1–38.

Buckner RL, Sepulcre J, Talukdar T, Krienen FM, Liu H, et al. 2009. Cortical hubs revealed by intrinsic functional connectivity: Mapping, assessment of stability, and relation to Alzheimer's disease. *J Neurosci* 29: 1860–1873.

Bullmore E, Sporns O. 2009. Complex brain networks: Graph theoretical analysis of structural and functional systems. *Nat Rev Neurosci* 10: 186–198.

Bullmore ET, Sporns O. 2012. The economy of brain network organization. *Nat Rev Neurosci* 13: 336–349.

Bullmore ET, Fletcher P, Jones PB. 2009. Why psychiatry can't afford to be neurophobic. *Br J Psychol* 194: 293–295.

Bullmore ET, Bassett DS. 2011. Brain graphs: Graphical models of the human brain connectome. *Annu Rev Clin Psychol* 7: 113–140.

Bushey D, Tononi G, Cirelli C. 2011. Sleep and synaptic homeostasis: Structural evidence in *Drosophila*. *Science* 332: 1576–1581.

Cabral J, Hugues E, Sporns O, Deco G. 2011. Role of local network oscillations in resting-state functional connectivity. *Neuroimage* 57: 130–139.

Cajal SR. 1995. *Histology of the Nervous System of Man and Vertebrates*. New York: Oxford University Press.

Cardona A, Saalfeld S, Preibisch S, Schmid B, Cheng A, et al. 2010. An integrated micro- and macroarchitectural analysis of the *Drosophila* brain by computer-assisted serial section electron microscopy. *PLoS Biol* 8: e1000502.

Catani M, Jones DK, ffytche DH. 2005. Perisylvian language networks of the human brain. *Ann Neurol* 57: 8–16.

Chang C, Glover GH. 2010. Time-frequency dynamics of resting-state brain connectivity measured with fMRI. *Neuroimage* 50: 81–98.

Changizi MA, Shimojo S. 2005. Parcellation and area-area connectivity as a function of neocortex size. *Brain Behav Evol* 66: 88–98.

Chen BL, Hall DH, Chklovskii DB. 2006. Wiring optimization can relate neuronal structure and function. *Proc Natl Acad Sci USA* 103: 4723–4728.

Chen JL, Nedivi E. 2010. Neuronal structural remodeling: Is it all about access? *Curr Opin Neurobiol* 20: 557–562.

Chen ZJ, He Y, Rosa-Neto P, Gong G, Evans AC. 2011. Age-related alterations in the modular organization of structural cortical network by using cortical thickness from MRI. *Neuroimage* 56: 235–245.

Chialvo DR. 2010. Emergent complex neural dynamics. *Nat Phys* 6: 744–750.

Chiang AS, Lin CY, Chuang CC, Chang HM, Hsieh CH, et al. 2011. Three-dimensional reconstruction of brain-wide wiring networks in *Drosophila* at single-cell resolution. *Curr Biol* 21: 1–11.

Chklovskii DB, Vitaladevuni S, Scheffer LK. 2010. Semi-automated reconstruction of neural circuits using electron microscopy. *Curr Opin Neurobiol* 20: 667–675.

Ch'ng YH, Reid RC. 2010. Cellular imaging of visual cortex reveals the spatial and functional organization of spontaneous activity. *Front Integr Neurosci* 4: 1.

Choe Y, Meyerich D, Kwon J, Miller DE, Chung JR, et al. 2011. Knife-edge scanning microscopy for connectomics research. In Proceedings of the International Joint Conference on Neural Networks, Piscataway, NJ, 2011. IEEE Press.

Chou YH, Spletter ML, Yaksi E, Leong JCS, Wilson RI, et al. 2010. Diversity and wiring variability of olfactory local interneurons in the *Drosophila* antennal lobe. *Nat Neurosci* 13: 439–449.

Chung JR, Sung C, Mayerich D, Kwon J, Miller DE, et al. 2011. Multiscale exploration of mouse brain microstructures using the knife-edge scanning microscope brain atlas. *Front Neuroinform* 5: 29.

Chung S, Courcot B, Sdika M, Moffat K, Rae C, et al. 2010. Bootstrap quantification of cardiac pulsation artifact in DTI. *Neuroimage* 49: 631–640.

Churchland PS, Sejnowski TJ. 1992. *The Computational Brain*. Cambridge: MIT Press.

Cirelli C. 2009. The genetic and molecular regulation of sleep: From fruit flies to humans. *Nat Rev Neurosci* 10: 549–560.

Clarke DD, Sokoloff L. 1999. Circulation and energy metabolism of the brain. In: Siegel GJ, Agranoff BW, Albers RW, Fisher SK, Uhler MD (eds.), *Basic Neurochemistry*, 6th ed., pp. 637–669. Philadelphia: Lippincott-Raven.

Cohen AL, Fair DA, Dosenbach NUF, Miezin FM, Dierker D, et al. 2008. Defining functional areas in individual human brains using resting state functional connectivity MRI. *Neuroimage* 41: 45–57.

Coleman JE, Nahmani M, Gavornik JP, Haslinger R, Heynen AJ, et al. 2010. Rapid structural remodelling of thalamocortical synapses parallels experience-dependent functional plasticity in mouse primary visual cortex. *J Neurosci* 30: 9670–9682.

Colizza V, Flammini A, Serrano MA, Vespignani A. 2006. Detecting rich-club ordering in complex networks. *Nat Phys* 2: 110–115.

Collins CE, Airey DC, Young NA, Leitch DB, Kaas JH. 2010. Neuron densities vary across and within cortical areas in primates. *Proc Natl Acad Sci USA* 107: 15927–15932.

Congdon E, Poldrack RA, Freimer NB. 2010. Neurocognitive phenotypes and genetic dissection of disorders of brain and behavior. *Neuron* 68: 218–230.

Conturo TE, Lori NF, Cull TS, Akbudak E, Snyder AZ, et al. 1999. Tracking neuronal fiber pathways in the living human brain. *Proc Natl Acad Sci USA* 96: 10422–10427.

Cook-Deegan RM. 1991. The Human Genome Project: The formation of federal policies in the United States, 1986–1990. In: Hanna KE (ed.), *Biomedical Politics*, pp. 99–168. Washington, DC: National Academy of Sciences.

Cook-Degan RM. 1994. *The Gene Wars: Science, Politics, and the Human Genome*. New York: Norton.

Costa LF, Travieso G. 2007. Exploring complex networks through random walks. *Phys Rev E Stat Nonlin Soft Matter Phys* 75: 016102.

Costa LF, Sporns O, Antiqueira L, Nunes M, Oliveira ON. 2007. Correlations between structure and random walk dynamics in directed complex networks. *Appl Phys Lett* 91: 054107.

Coveney PV, Fowler PW. 2005. Modelling biological complexity: A physical scientist's perspective. *J R Soc Interface* 22: 267–280.

Crick F. 1984. Neurobiology: Memory and molecular turnover. *Nature* 312: 101.

Crofts JJ, Higham DJ, Bosnell R, Jbabdi S, Matthews PM, et al. 2011. Network analysis detects changes in the contralesional hemisphere following stroke. *Neuroimage* 54: 161–169.

Cuntz H, Forstner F, Borst A, Häusser M. 2010. One rule to grow them all: A general theory of neuronal branching and its practical application. *PLoS Comput Biol* 6: e1000877.

Curcio CA, Sloan KR, Packer O, Hendrickson AE, Kalina RE. 1987. Distribution of cones in human and monkey retina: Individual variability and radial asymmetry. *Science* 236: 579–582.

da Costa NM, Martin KAC. 2010. Whose cortical column would that be? *Front Neuroanat* 4: 16.

Dada JO, Mendes P. 2011. Multi-scale modelling and simulation in systems biology. *Integr Biol* 3: 86–96.

Damoiseaux JS, Rombouts SARB, Barkhof F, Scheltens P, Stam CJ, et al. 2006. Consistent resting-state networks across healthy subjects. *Proc Natl Acad Sci USA* 103: 13848–13853.

Damoiseaux JS, Greicius MD. 2009. Greater than the sum of its parts: A review of studies combining structural connectivity and resting-state functional connectivity. *Brain Struct Funct* 213: 525–533.

Das A, Gilbert CD. 1995. Long-range horizontal connections and their role in cortical reorganization revealed by optical recording of cat primary visual cortex. *Nature* 375: 780–784.

Dauguet J, Peled S, Berezovskii V, Delzescaux T, Warfield SK, et al. 2007. Comparison of fiber tracts derived from in-vivo DTI tractography with 3D histological neural tract tracer reconstruction on a macaque brain. *Neuroimage* 27: 530–538.

Deacon TW. 1990. Rethinking mammalian brain evolution. *Am Zool* 30: 629–705.

Deco G, Jirsa V, McIntosh AR, Sporns O, Kötter R. 2009. Key role of coupling, delay, and noise in resting brain fluctuations. *Proc Natl Acad Sci USA* 106: 10302–10307.

Deco G, Corbetta M. 2011. The dynamical balance of the brain at rest. *Neuroscientist* 17: 107–123.

Deco G, Jirsa VK, McIntosh AR. 2011. Emerging concepts for the dynamical organization of resting-state activity in the brain. *Nat Rev Neurosci* 12: 43–56.

De Felipe J. 2010. From the connectome to the synaptome: An epic love story. *Science* 330: 1198–1201.

Dejerine J. 1895. *Anatomie des Centres Nerveux*. Paris: Rueff.

De Luca M, Beckmann CF, De Stefano N, Matthews PM, Smith SM. 2006. fMRI resting state networks define distinct modes of long-distance interactions in the human brain. *Neuroimage* 29: 1359–1367.

Denk W, Briggman KL, Helmstaedter M. 2012. Structural neurobiology: Missing link to a mechanistic understanding of neural computation. *Nat Rev Neurosci* doi: 10.1038/nrn3169.

Denk W, Horstmann H. 2004. Serial block-face scanning electron microscopy to reconstruct three-dimensional tissue nanostructure. *PLoS Biol* 2: e329.

de Pasquale F, Della Penna S, Snyder AZ, Lewis C, Mantini D, et al. 2010. Temporal dynamics of spontaneous MEG activity in brain networks. *Proc Natl Acad Sci USA* 107: 6040–6045.

Desai M, Kahn I, Knoblich U, Bernstein J, Atallah H, et al. 2011. Mapping brain networks in awake mice using combined optical neural control and fMRI. *J Neurophysiol* 105: 1393–1405.

De Schutter E. 2008. Why are computational neuroscience and systems biology so separate? *PLoS Comput Biol* 4: e1000078.

Dong HW. 2007. *The Allen Atlas: A Digital Brain Atlas of C57BL/6J Male Mouse*. Hoboken, NJ: Wiley.

Donohue DE, Ascoli GA. 2011. Automated reconstruction of neuronal morphology: An overview. *Brain Res Brain Res Rev* 67: 94–102.

Doucet G, Naveau M, Petit L, Delcroix N, Zago L, et al. 2011. Brain activity at rest: A multiscale hierarchical functional organization. *J Neurophysiol* 105: 2753–2763.

Douglas RJ, Martin KAC, Whitteridge D. 1989. A canonical microcircuit for neocortex. *Neural Comput* 1: 480–488.

Douglas RJ, Martin KAC. 2004. Neuronal circuits of the neocortex. *Annu Rev Neurosci* 27: 419–451.

Douglas RJ, Martin KAC. 2011. What's black and white about the grey matter? *Neuroinformatics* 9: 167–179.

Doyle DA, Cabral JM, Pfuetzner RA, Kuo A, Gulbis JM, et al. 1998. The structure of the potassium channel: Molecular basis of K^+ conduction and selectivity. *Science* 280: 69–77.

Drzezga A, Becker JA, van Dijk KRA, Sreenivasan A, Talukdar T, et al. 2011. Neuronal dysfunction and disconnection of cortical hubs in non-demented subjects with elevated amyloid burden. *Brain* 134: 1635–1646.

Durbin RM, Abecasis GR, Altshuler DL, Auton A, Brooks LD, et al. 2010. A map of human genome variation from population-scale sequencing. *Nature* 467: 1061–1073.

Ecker AS, Berens P, Keliris GA, Bethge M, Logothetis NK, et al. 2010. Decorrelated neuronal firing in cortical microcircuits. *Science* 327: 584–587.

Editorial. 2010. A critical look at connectomics. *Nature Neuroscience* 13: 1441.

Ehlers MD. 2003. Activity level controls postsynaptic composition and signaling via the ubiquitin–proteasome system. *Nat Neurosci* 6: 231–242.

Eickhoff SB, Bzdok D, Laird AR, Roski C, Caspers S, et al. 2011. Co-activation patterns distinguish cortical modules, their connectivity and functional differentiation. *Neuroimage* 57: 938–949.

Estrada E, Rodriguez-Velázquez JA. 2005. Subgraph centrality in complex networks. *Phys Rev E Stat Nonlin Soft Matter Phys* 71: 056103.

Exner S. 1894 *Entwurf zu einer physiologischen Erklärung der psychischen Erscheinungen.* Leipzig: Franz Deuticke.

Fair DA, Cohen AL, Power JD, Dosenbach NUF, Church JA, et al. 2009. Functional brain networks develop from a "local to distributed" organization. *PLoS Comput Biol* 5: e1000381.

Fan Y, Shi F, Smith JK, Lin W, Gilmore JH, et al. 2011. Brain anatomical networks in early human brain development. *Neuroimage* 54: 1862–1871.

Feinberg DA, Moeller S, Smith SM, Auerbach E, Ramanna S, et al. 2010. Multiplexed echo planar imaging for sub-second whole brain fMRI and fast diffusion imaging. *PLoS ONE* 5: e15710.

Feldt S, Bonifazi P, Cossart R. 2011. Dissecting functional connectivity of neuronal microcurcuits: Experimental and theoretical insights. *Trends Neurosci* 34: 225–236.

Felleman DJ, van Essen DC. 1991. Distributed hierarchical processing in the primate cerebral cortex. *Cereb Cortex* 1: 1–47.

Ferrarelli F, Massimini M, Sarasso S, Casali A, Riedner BA, et al. 2010. Breakdown in cortical effective connectivity during midazolam-induced loss of consciousness. *Proc Natl Acad Sci USA* 107: 2681–2686.

Fields RD. 2010. *The Other Brain.* New York: Simon and Schuster.

Fox MD, Raichle M. 2007. Spontaneous fluctuations in brain activity observed with functional magnetic resonance imaging. *Nat Rev Neurosci* 8: 700–711.

Fox PT, Lancaster JL. 2002. Mapping context and content: The BrainMap model. *Nat Rev Neurosci* 3: 319–321.

Fransson P, Marrelec G. 2008. The precuneus/posterior cingulate cortex plays a pivotal role in the default mode network: Evidence from a partial correlation network analysis. *Neuroimage* 42: 1178–1184.

French L, Pavlidis P. 2011. Relationships between gene expression and brain wiring in the adult rodent brain. *PLoS Comput Biol* 7: e1001049.

French L, Tan PPC, Pavlidis P. 2011. Large-scale analysis of gene expression and connectivity in the rodent brain: Insights through data integration. *Front Neuroinf* 5: 12.

Freud S. 1966. Project for a scientific psychology. In Strachey J (ed. and trans.), *The Standard Edition of the Complete Psychological Works of Sigmund Freud*, vol. 1, pp. 295–397. London: Hogarth Press.

Friston KJ, Harrison L, Penny W. 2003. Dynamic causal modelling. *Neuroimage* 19: 1273–1302.

Friston KJ. 2009. Modalities, modes, and models in functional neuroimaging. *Science* 326: 399–403.

Friston KJ. 2011. Functional and effective connectivity: A review. *Brain Connectivity* 1: 13–36.

Friston KJ, Li B, Daunizeau J, Stephan KE. 2011. Network discovery with DCM. *Neuroimage* 56: 1202–1221.

Galbraith CG, Galbraith JA. 2011. Super-resolution microscopy at a glance. *J Cell Sci* 124: 1607–1611.

Ganmor E, Segev R, Schneidman E. 2011. The architecture of functional interaction networks in the retina. *J Neurosci* 23: 3044–3054.

Gastner MT, Newman MEJ. 2006. The spatial structure of networks. *Eur Phys J B* 49: 247–252.

Gerhard S, Daducci A, Lemkaddem A, Meuli R, Thiran JP, et al. 2011. The Connectome Viewer Toolkit: An open source framework to manage, analyze, and visualize connectomes. *Front Neuroinf* 5: 3.

Ghosh A, Rho Y, McIntosh AR, Kötter R, Jirsa VK. 2008. Noise during rest enables the exploration of the brain's dynamic repertoire. *PLoS Comput Biol* 4: e1000196.

Gilbert CD, Sigman M, Crist RE. 2001. The neural basis of perceptual learning. *Neuron* 31: 681–697.

Giot L, Bader JS, Brouwer C, Chauduri A, Kuang B, et al. 2003. A protein interaction map of *Drosophila* melanogaster. *Science* 302: 1727–1736.

Glahn DC, Thompson PM, Blangero J. 2007. Neuroimaging endophenotypes: Strategies for finding genes influencing brain structure and function. *Hum Brain Mapp* 28: 488–501.

Glahn DC, Winkler AM, Kochunov P, Almasy L, Duggirala R, et al. 2010. Genetic control over the resting brain. *Proc Natl Acad Sci USA* 107: 1223–1228.

Glasser MF, Van Essen DC. 2011. Mapping human cortical areas in vivo based on myelin content as revealed by T1- and T2-weighted MRI. *J Neurosci* 31: 11597–11616.

Glissen E, Zilles K. 1995. The relative volume of the primary visual cortex and its intersubject variability among humans: A new morphometric strudy. *C.R. Acad Sci Paris* 320: 897–902.

Goaillard JM, Taylor AL, Schulz DJ, Marder E. 2009. Functional consequences of animal-to-animal variation in circuit parameters. *Nat Neurosci* 12: 1424–1430.

Goldschmidt R. 1908. Das Nervensystem von Ascaris lumbricoides und megalocephala: Ein Versuch, in den Aufbau eines einfachen Nervensystems einzudringen. *Erster Teil Zeitschrift Wiss Zool* 90: 73–136.

Gong G, He Y, Concha L, Lebel C, Gross DW, et al. 2009. Mapping anatomical connectivity patterns of human cerebral cortex using in vivo diffusion tensor imaging tractography. *Cereb Cortex* 19: 524–536.

Granovetter MS. 1973. The strength of weak ties. *Am J Sociol* 78: 1360–1380.

Grefkes C, Fink GR. 2011. Reorganization of cerebral networks after stroke: New insights from neuroimaging with connectivity approaches. *Brain* 134: 1264–1276.

Greicius MD, Krasnow B, Reiss AL, Menon V. 2003. Functional connectivity in the resting brain: A network analysis of the default mode hypothesis. *Proc Natl Acad Sci USA* 100: 253–258.

Greicius MD, Supekar K, Menon V, Dougherty RF. 2009. Resting state functional connectivity reflects structural connectivity in the default mode network. *Cereb Cortex* 19: 72–78.

Grigg O, Grady CL. 2010. Task-related effects on the temporal and spatial dynamics of resting-state functional connectivity in the default network. *PLoS ONE* 5: e13311.

Guimerà R, Mossa S, Turtschi A, Amaral LAN. 2005. The worldwide air transportation network: Anomalous centrality, community structure, and cities' global roles. *Proc Natl Acad Sci USA* 102: 7794–7799.

Guye M, Bettus G, Bartolomei F, Cozzone PJ. 2010. Graph theoretical analysis of structural and functional connectivity MRI in normal and pathological brain networks. *Magn Reson Mater Phy* 23: 409–421.

Hadjieconomou D, Rotkopf S, Alexandre C, Bell DM, Dickson BJ, et al. 2011. Flybow: Genetic multicolor cell labeling for neural circuit analysis in *Drosophila* melanogaster. *Nat Methods* 8: 260–266.

Hagmann P. 2005. From Diffusion MRI to Brain Connectomics. PhD Thesis, Ecole Polytechnique Fédérale de Lausanne, Lausanne, France.

Hagmann P, Kurant M, Gigandet X, Thiran P, Wedeen VJ, et al. 2007. Mapping human whole-brain structural networks with diffusion MRI. *PLoS ONE* 2: e597.

Hagmann P, Cammoun L, Gigandet X, Meuli R, Honey CJ, et al. 2008. Mapping the structural core of human cerebral cortex. *PLoS Biol* 6: e159.

Hagmann P, Cammoun L, Gigandet X, Gerhard S, Grant PE, et al. 2010a. MR connectomics: Principles and challenges. *J Neurosci Methods* 194: 34–45.

Hagmann P, Sporns O, Madan N, Cammoun L, Pienaar R, et al. 2010b. White matter maturation reshapes structural connectivity in the late developing human brain. *Proc Natl Acad Sci USA* 107: 19067–19072.

Hall DH, Russell RL. 1991. The posterior nervous system of the nematode *Caenorhabditis elegans*: Serial reconstruction of identified neurons and complete pattern of synaptic interactions. *J Neurosci* 11: 1–22.

Hama H, Kurokawa H, Kawano H, Ando R, Shimogori T, et al. 2011. Scale: A chemical approach for fluorescence imaging and reconstruction of transparent mouse brain. *Nature Neurosci* 14: 1481–1488.

Hampel S, Chung P, McKellar CE, Hall D, Looger LL, et al. 2011. *Drosophila* Brainbow: A recombinase-based fluorescence labeling technique to subdivide neural expression patterns. *Nat Methods* 8: 253–259.

Harris KM, Perry E, Bourne J, Feinberg M, Ostroff L, et al. 2006. Uniform serial sectioning for transmission electron microscopy. *J Neurosci* 26: 12101–12103.

Hasson U, Nir Y, Levy I, Fuhrmann G, Malach R. 2004. Intersubject synchronization of cortical activity during natural vision. *Science* 303: 1634–1640.

Haxby JV, Gobbini MI, Furey ML, Ishai A, Schouten JL, et al. 2001. Distributed and overlapping representations of faces and objects in ventral temporal cortex. *Science* 293: 2425–2430.

Hayasaka S, Laurienti PJ. 2010. Comparison of characteristics between region- and voxel-based network analyses in resting-state fMRI data. *Neuroimage* 50: 499–508.

Haynes JD, Rees G. 2005. Predicting the stream of consciousness from activity in human visual cortex. *Curr Biol* 15: 1301–1307.

Haynes JD, Rees G. 2006. Decoding mental states from brain activity in humans. *Nat Rev Neurosci* 7: 523–534.

He Y, Chen ZJ, Evans AC. 2007. Small-world anatomical networks in the human brain revealed by cortical thickness from MRI. *Cereb Cortex* 17: 2407–2419.

Helmstaedter M, Briggman KL, Denk W. 2011. High-accuracy neurite reconstruction for high-throughput neuroanatomy. *Nat Neurosci* 14: 1081–1088.

Helmstaedter M, Mitra PP. 2012. Computational methods and challenges for large-scale circuit mapping. *Curr Opin Neurobiol* 22: 162–169.

Herculano-Houzel S, Mota B, Wong P, Kaas JH. 2010. Connectivity-driven white matter scaling and folding in primate cerebral cortex. *Proc Natl Acad Sci USA* 107: 19008–19013.

Hilbert M, López P. 2011. The world's technological capacity to store, communicate, and compute information. *Science* 332: 60–65.

Hilgetag CC, Burns GA, O'Neill MA, Scannell JW, Young MP. 2000. Anatomical connectivity defines the organization of clusters of cortical areas in the macaque monkey and the cat. *Phil Trans R Soc B* 355: 91–110.

Hilgetag CC, Kaiser M. 2004. Clustered organization of cortical connectivity. *Neuroinformatics* 2: 353–360.

Hofer SB, Mrsic-Flogel TD, Bonhoeffer T, Hübener M. 2009. Experience leaves a lasting structural trace in cortical circuits. *Nature* 457: 313–317.

Holtmaat AJGD, Trachtenberg JT, Wilbrecht L, Shepherd GM, Zhang X, et al. 2005. Transient and persistent dendritic spines in the neocortex in vivo. *Neuron* 45: 279–291.

Holtmaat A, Svoboda K. 2009. Experience-dependent structural synaptic plasticity in the mammalian brain. *Nat Rev Neurosci* 10: 647–658.

Honey CJ, Kötter R, Breakspear M, Sporns O. 2007. Network structure of cerebral cortex shapes functional connectivity on multiple time scales. *Proc Natl Acad Sci USA* 104: 10240–10245.

Honey CJ, Sporns O, Cammoun L, Gigandet X, Thiran JP, et al. 2009. Predicting human resting-state functional connectivity from structural connectivity. *Proc Natl Acad Sci USA* 106: 2035–2040.

Honey CJ, Thivierge JP, Sporns O. 2010. Can structure predict function in the human brain? *Neuroimage* 52: 766–776.

Hood L, Heath JR, Phelps ME, Lin B. 2004. Systems biology and new technologies enable predictive and preventative medicine. *Science* 306: 640–643.

Hunter PJ, Borg TK. 2003. Integration from proteins to organs: The Physiome Project. *Nat Rev Mol Cell Biol* 4: 237–243.

Hutchison RM, Leung LS, Mirsattari SM, Gati JS, Menon RS, et al. 2011. Resting-state networks in the macaque at 7T. *Neuroimage* 56: 1546–1555.

Hyman SE. 2010. The diagnosis of mental disorders: The problem of reification. *Annu Rev Clin Psychol* 6: 155–179.

Ideker T, Galitski T, Hood L. 2001. A new approach to decoding life: Systems biology. *Annu Rev Genomics Hum Genet* 2: 343–372.

Insel T, Cuthbert B, Garvey M, Heinssen R, Pine DS, et al. 2010. Research domain criteria (RDoC): Toward a new classification framework for research on mental disorders. *Am J Psychiatry* 167: 748–751.

Irimia A, Chambers MC, Torgerson CM, Filippou M, Hovda DA, et al. 2012. Patient-tailored connectomics visualization for the assessment of white matter atrophy in traumatic brain injury. *Front Neurol* 3: 10.

Iturria-Medina Y, Canales-Rodriguez EJ, Melie-Garcia L, Valdes-Hernandez PA, Martinez-Montes E, et al. 2007. Characterizing brain anatomical connections using diffusion weighted MRI and graph theory. *Neuroimage* 36: 645–660.

Iturria-Medina Y, Sotero RC, Canales-Rodriguez EJ, Aleman-Gomez Y, Melie-Garcia L. 2008. Studying the human brain anatomical network via diffusion-weighted MRI and graph theory. *Neuroimage* 40: 1064–1076.

Jain V, Seung HS, Turaga SS. 2010. Machines that learn to segment images: A crucial technology for connectomics. *Curr Opin Neurobiol* 20: 653–666.

Jaume S, Knobe K, Newton R, Schlimbach F, Blower M, et al. 2011. A multi-scale parallel computing architecture for automated segmentation of the brain connectome. *IEEE Trans Biomed Eng* 99: 1.

Jbabdi S, Johansen-Berg H. 2011. Tractography: Where do we go from here? *Brain Connectivity* 1: 169–183.

Jeong WK, Beyer J, Hadwiger M, Blue R, Law C, et al. 2010. Scecrett and NeuroTrace: Interactive visualization and analysis tools for large-scale neuroscience data sets. *IEEE Comput Graph Appl* 30: 58–70.

Jiang Y, Johnson GA. 2011. Microscopic diffusion tensor atlas of the mouse brain. *Neuroimage* 56: 1235–1243.

Jirsa VK. 2004. Connectivity and dynamics of neural information processing. *Neuroinformatics* 2: 183–204.

Jirsa VK, McIntosh AR. 2007. *Handbook of Brain Connectivity*. New York: Springer.

Jirsa VK, Sporns O, Breakspear M, Deco G, McIntosh AR. 2010. Towards the virtual brain: Network modeling of the intact and the damaged brain. *Arch Ital Biol* 148: 189–205.

Johansen-Berg H, Behrens TE, Robson MD, Drobnjak I, Rushworth MF, et al. 2004. Changes in connectivity profiles define functionally distinct regions in human medial frontal cortex. *Proc Natl Acad Sci USA* 101: 13335–13340.

Johansen-Berg H, Behrens TEJ, Sillery E, Ciccarelli O, Thompson AJ, et al. 2005. Functional–anatomical validation and individual variation of diffusion tractography-based segmentation of the human thalamus. *Cereb Cortex* 15: 31–39.

Johansen-Berg H, Della-Maggiore V, Behrens TEJ, Smith SM, Paus T. 2007. Integrity of white matter in the corpus callosum correlates with bimanual co-ordination skills. *Neuroimage* 36(Suppl. 2): T16–T21.

Johansen-Berg H, Rushworth MFS. 2009. Using diffusion imaging to study human connectional anatomy. *Annu Rev Neurosci* 32: 75–94.

Johansen-Berg H, Behrens TEJ, eds. 2009. *Diffusion MRI: From Quantitative Measurement to in Vivo Neuroanatomy*. Amsterdam: Academic Press.

Johansen-Berg H, Scholz J, Stagg CJ. 2010. Relevance of structural brain connectivity to learning and recovery from stroke. *Front Syst Neurosci* 4: 146.

Johnston JM, Vaishnavi SN, Smyth MD, Zhang D, He BJ, et al. 2008. Loss of resting interhemispheric functional connectivity after complete section of the corpus callosum. *J Neurosci* 28: 6453–6458.

Joyce AR, Palsson BO. 2007. The model organism as a system: Integrating "omics" data sets. *Nat Rev Mol Cell Biol* 7: 198–210.

Kaiser M, Hilgetag CC. 2006. Nonoptimal component placement, but short processing paths, due to long-distance projections in neural systems. *PLoS Comput Biol* 2: e95.

Kaiser M. 2011. Tutorial in connectome analysis: Topological and spatial features of brain networks. *Neuroimage* 57: 892–907.

Kamada T, Kawai S. 1989. An algorithm for drawing general undirected graphs. *Inf Process Lett* 31: 7–15.

Kanai R, Bahrami B, Rees G. 2010. Human parietal cortex structure predicts individual differences in perceptual rivalry. *Curr Biol* 20: 1626–1630.

Kanai R, Rees G. 2011. The structural basis of inter-individual differences in human behaviour and cognition. *Nat Rev Neurosci* 12: 231–242.

Kasparian G, Brugger PC, Weber M, Krssák M, Krampl E, et al. 2008. In utero tractography of fetal white matter development. *Neuroimage* 43: 213–224.

Kasthuri N, Hayworth K, Lichtman J, Erdman N, Ackerley CA. 2007. New technique for ultra-thin serial brain section imaging using scanning electron microscopy. *Microsc Microanal* 13: 26–27.

Kasthuri N, Lichtman JW. 2010. Neurocartography. *Neuropsychopharmacology* 35: 342–343.

Keck T, Mrsic-Flogel TD, Afonso MV, Eysel UT, Bonhoeffer T, et al. 2008. Massive restructuring of neuronal circuits during functional reorganization of adult visual cortex. *Nat Neurosci* 11: 1162–1167.

Kell DB, Oliver SG. 2004. Here is the evidence, now what is the hypothesis? The complementary roles of inductive and hypothesis-driven science in the post-genomic era. *Bioessays* 26: 99–105.

Kendler KS, Aggen SH, Knudsen GP, Røysamb E, Neale MC, et al. 2011. The structure of genetic and environmental risk factors for syndromal and subsyndromal common DSM-IV axis I and all axis II disorders. *Am J Psychiatry* 168: 29–39.

Khanna PC, Poliakov AV, Ishak GE, Poliachik SL, Friedman SD, et al. 2011. Preserved interhemispheric functional connectivity in a case of corpus callosum agenesis. *Neuroradiology* 54: 177–179.

Kinnunen KM, Greenwood R, Powell JH, Leech R, Hawkins PC, et al. 2011. White matter damage and cognitive impairment after traumatic brain injury. *Brain* 134: 449–463.

Kitano H. 2001. *Foundations of Systems Biology*. Cambridge: MIT Press.

Kitano H. 2002. Systems biology: A brief overview. *Science* 295: 1662–1664.

Kleinfeld D, Bharioke A, Blinder P, Bock DD, Briggman KL, et al. 2011. Large-scale automated histology in the pursuit of connectomes. *J Neurosci* 31: 16125–16138.

Knösche TR, Tittgemeyer M. 2011. The role of long-range connectivity for the characterization of the functional–anatomical organization of the cortex. *Front Syst Neurosci* 5: 58.

Knott G, Marchman H, Wall D, Lich B. 2008. Serial section scanning electron microscopy of adult brain tissue using focused ion beam milling. *J Neurosci* 28: 2959–2964.

Ko H, Hofer SB, Pichler B, Buchanan KA, Sjöström PJ, et al. 2011. Functional specificity of local synaptic connections in neocortical networks. *Nature* 473: 87–91.

Kötter R. 2004. Online retrieval, processing, and visualization of primate connectivity data from the CoCoMac database. *Neuroinformatics* 2: 127–144.

Kötter R. 2007. Anatomical concepts of brain connectivity. In: Jirsa VK, McIntosh AR (eds), *Handbook of Brain Connectivity*, pp. 149–167. Berlin: Springer.

Krishnan A, Zbilut JP, Tomita M, Giuliani A. 2008. Proteins as networks: Usefulness of graph theory in protein science. *Curr Protein Pept Sci* 9: 28–38.

Krubitzer L. 2007. The magnificent compromise: Cortical field evolution in mammals. *Neuron* 56: 201–208.

Kurth F, Eickhoff SB, Schleicher A, Hoemke L, Zilles K, et al. 2010. Cytoarchitecture and probabilistic maps of the human posterior insular cortex. *Cereb Cortex* 20: 1448–1461.

Kurzweil R. 2000. *The Age of Spiritual Machines*. New York: Penguin Books.

Laird AR, Lancaster JL, Fox PT. 2005. BrainMap: The social evolution of a human brain mapping database. *Neuroinformatics* 3: 65–78.

Laughlin SB, Sejnowski TJ. 2003. Communication in neuronal networks. *Science* 301: 1870–1874.

Laureys S, Owen AM, Schiff ND. 2004. Brain function in coma, vegetative state, and related disorders. *Lancet Neurol* 3: 537–546.

Lazer D, Pentland A, Adamic L, Aral S, Barabasi AL, et al. 2009. Life in the network: The coming age of computational social science. *Science* 323: 721–723.

Le Bihan D, Mangin JF, Poupon C, Clark CA, Pappata S, et al. 2001. Diffusion tensor imaging: Concepts and applications. *J Magn Reson Imaging* 13: 534–546.

Le Bihan D. 2003. Looking into the functional architecture of the brain with diffusion MRI. *Nat Rev Neurosci* 4: 469–480.

Lee JH, Durand R, Gradinaru V, Zhang F, Goshen I, et al. 2010. Global and local fMRI signals driven by neurons defined optogenetically by type and wiring. *Nature* 465: 788–792.

Lee JH. 2011. Tracing activity across the whole brain neural network with optogenetic functional magnetic resonance imaging. *Front Neuroinform* 5: 21.

Lee WCA, Huang H, Feng G, Sanes JR, Brown EN, et al. 2005. Dynamic remodeling of dendritic arbors in GABAergic interneurons of adult visual cortex. *PLoS Biol* 4: e29.

Lee WCA, Reid RC. 2011. Specificity and randomness: Structure–function relationships in neural circuits. *Curr Opin Neurobiol* 21: 801–807.

Leech R, Braga R, Sharp DJ. 2012. Echoes of the brain within the posterior cingulate cortex. *J Neurosci* 32: 215–222.

Leergaard TB, White NS, de Crespigny A, Bolstad I, D'Arceuil H, et al. 2010. Quantitative histological validation of diffusion MRI fiber orientation distributions in the rat brain. *PLoS ONE* 5: e8595.

Legenstein R, Maass W. 2011. Branch-specific plasticity enables self-organization of non-linear computation in single neurons. *J Neurosci* 31: 10787–10802.

Lehmann D, Ozaki H, Pal I. 1987. EEG alpha map series: Brain micro-states by space-oriented adaptive segmentation. *Electroencephalogr Clin Neurophysiol* 67: 271–288.

Lehmann D. 1990. Brain electric microstates and cognition: The atoms of thought. In: John ER (ed), *Machinery of the Mind*, pp. 209–224. Boston: Birkhäuser.

Lein ES, Hawrylycz MJ, Ao N, Ayres M, Bensinger A, et al. 2007. Genome-wide atlas of gene expression in the adult mouse brain. *Nature* 445: 168–176.

Lerch JP, Worsley K, Shaw WP, Greenstein DK, Lenroot RK, et al. 2006. Mapping anatomical correlations across cerebral cortex (MACACC) using cortical thickness from MRI. *Neuroimage* 31: 993–1003.

Lewis CM, Baldassare A, Committeri G, Romani GL, Corbetta M. 2009. Learning sculpts the spontaneous activity of the resting human brain. *Proc Natl Acad Sci USA* 106: 17558–17563.

Li A, Gong H, Zhang B, Wang Q, Yan C, et al. 2010a. Micro-optical sectioning tomography to obtain a high-resolution atlas of the mouse brain. *Science* 330: 1401–1408.

Li L, Taskic B, Micheva KD, Ivanov VM, Spletter ML, et al. 2010b. Visualizing the distribution of synapses from individual neurons in the mouse brain. *PLoS ONE* 5: e11503.

Li S, Armstrong CM, Bertin N, Ge H, Milstein S, et al. 2004. A map of the interactome network of the metazoan C. elegans. *Science* 303: 540–543.

Li Y, Liu Y, Li J, Qin W, Li K, et al. 2009. Brain anatomical network and intelligence. *PLoS Comput Biol* 5: e1000395.

Lichtman JW, Livet J, Sanes JR. 2008. A technicolour approach to the connectome. *Nat Rev Neurosci* 9: 417–422.

Lichtman JW, Denk W. 2011. The big and the small: Challenges of imaging the brain's circuits. *Science* 334: 618–623.

Lieberman-Aiden E, van Berkum NL, Williams L, Imakaev M, Ragoczy T, et al. 2009. Comprehensive mapping of long-range interactions reveals folding principles of the human genome. *Science* 326: 289–293.

Lisman JE. 1985. A mechanism for memory storage insensitive to molecular turnover: A bistable autophoshorylating kinase. *Proc Natl Acad Sci USA* 82: 3055–3057.

Liu ZW, Faraguna U, Cirelli C, Tononi G, Gao XB. 2010. Direct evidence for wake-related increases and sleep-related decreases in synaptic strength in rodent cortex. *J Neurosci* 30: 8671–8675.

Livet J, Weissman TA, Kang H, Draft RW, Lu J, et al. 2007. Transgenic strategies for combinatorial expression of fluorescent proteins in the nervous system. *Nature* 450: 56–62.

London M, Häusser M. 2005. Dendritic computation. *Annu Rev Neurosci* 28: 503–532.

Long F, Peng H, Liu X, Kim SK, Myers E. 2008. A 3D digital atlas of *C. elegans* and its application to single-cell analyses. *Nat Methods* 6: 667–672.

Lu J, Tapia JC, White OL, Lichtman JW. 2009. The interscutularis muscle connectome. *PLoS Biol* 7: e1000032.

Lu J. 2011. Neuronal tracing for connectomic studies. *Neuroinformatics* 9: 159–166.

Mantini D, Gerits A, Nelissen K, Durand JB, Joly O, et al. 2011. Default mode of brain function in monkeys. *J Neurosci* 31: 12954–12962.

Marcus DS, Harwell J, Olsen T, Hodge M, Glasser MF, et al. 2011. Informatics and data mining tools and strategies for the Human Connectome Project. *Front Neuroinf* 5: 4.

Marder E. 2011. Variability, compensation, and modulation in neurons and circuits. *Proc Natl Acad Sci USA* 108: 15542–15548.

Marder E, Taylor AL. 2011. Multiple models to capture the variability in biological neurons and networks. *Nat Neurosci* 14: 133–138.

Markov NT, Misery P, Falchier A, Lamy C, Vezoli J, et al. 2011. Weight consistency specifies regularities of macaque cortical networks. *Cereb Cortex* 21: 1254–1272.

Markram H. 2006. The Blue Brain Project. *Nat Rev Neurosci* 7: 153–160.

Mars RB, Jbabdi S, Sallet J, O'Reilly JX, Croxson PL, et al. 2011. Diffusion-weighted imaging tractography-based parcellation of the human parietal cortex and comparison with human and macaque resting-state functional connectivity. *J Neurosci* 31: 4087–4100.

Massimini M, Ferrarelli F, Huber R, Esser SK, Singh H, et al. 2005. Breakdown of cortical effective connectivity during sleep. *Science* 309: 2228–2232.

Mayerich D, Abbott LC, McCormick BH. 2008. Knife-edge scanning microscopy for imaging and reconstruction of three-dimensional anatomical structures of the mouse brain. *J Microsc* 231: 134–143.

McCulloch WS. 1944. The functional organization of the cerebral cortex. *Physiol Rev* 24: 390–407.

McCulloch WS, Pitts W. 1948. The statistical organization of nervous activity. *Biometrics* 4: 91–99.

McIntosh AR, Grady CL, Ungerleider LG, Haxby JV, Rapoport SI, et al. 1994. Network analysis of cortical visual pathways mapped with PET. *J Neurosci* 14: 655–666.

Menon V. 2011. Large-scale brain networks and psychopathology: A unifying triple network model. *Trends Cogn Sci* 15: 483–506.

Merchán-Pérez A, Rodriguez JR, Alonso-Nanclares L, Schertel A, De Felipe J. 2009. Counting synapses using FIB/SEM microscopy: A true revolution for ultrastructural volume reconstruction. *Front Neuroanat* 3: 18.

Merkle RC. 1989. Large Scale Analysis of Neural Structures. Xerox PARC technical report: CSL-89–10 November 1989, [P89–00173].

Mesulam M. 2005. Imaging connectivity in the human cerebral cortex: The next frontier? *Ann Neurol* 57: 5–7.

Meunier D, Lambiotte R, Fornito A, Ersche KD, Bullmore ET. 2009. Hierarchical modularity in human brain functional networks. *Front Neuroinf* 3: 37.

Meynert T. 1885. *Psychiatry: A Clinical Treatise on Diseases of the Fore-Brain*. New York: Putnam's.

Micheva KD, Smith SK. 2007. Array tomography: A new tool for imaging the molecular architecture and ultrastructure of neural circuits. *Neuron* 55: 25–36.

Micheva KD, Busse B, Weiler NC, O'Rourke N, Smith SJ. 2010. Single-synapse analysis of a diverse synapse population: Proteomic imaging methods and markers. *Neuron* 68: 639–653.

Micheva KD, Bruchez MP. 2012. The gain in brain: Novel imaging techniques and multiplexed proteomic imaging of brain tissue architecture. *Curr Opin Neurobiol* 22: 94–100.

Miller KL, Stagg CJ, Douaud G, Jbabdi S, Smith SM, et al. 2011. Diffusion imaging of whole, post-mortem human brains on a clinical MRI scanner. *Neuroimage* 57: 167–181.

Mishchenko Y, Hu T, Spacek J, Mendenhall J, Harris KM, et al. 2010. Ultrastructural analysis of hippocampal neuropil from the connectomics perspective. *Neuron* 67: 1009–1020.

Mishchenko Y. 2011. Reconstruction of complete connectivity matrix for connectomics by sampling neural connectivity with fluorescent synaptic markers. *J Neurosci Methods* 196: 289–302.

Missiuro PV, Liu K, Zou L, Ross BC, Zhao G, et al. 2009. Information flow analysis of interactome networks. *PLoS Comput Biol* 5: e1000350.

Modha DS, Ananthanarayanan R, Esser SK, Ndirango A, Sherbondy AJ, et al. 2011. Cognitive computing. *Commun ACM* 54(8): 62–71.

Mori S, Crain BJ, Chacko VP, van Zijl PCM. 1999. Three-dimensional tracking of axonal projections in the brain by magnetic resonance imaging. *Ann Neurol* 45: 265–269.

Mountcastle VB. 1997. The columnar organization of the neocortex. *Brain* 120: 701–722.

Moussa MN, Vechlekar CD, Burdette JH, Steen MR, Hugenschmidt CE, et al. 2011. Changes in cognitive state alter human functional brain networks. *Front Hum Neurosci* 5: 83.

Musso F, Brinkmeyer J, Mobascher A, Warbrick T, Winterer G. 2010. Spontaneous brain activity and EEG microstates: A novel EEG/fMRI analysis approach to explore resting-state networks. *Neuroimage* 52: 1149–1161.

Nelson SM, Cohen AL, Power JD, Wig GS, Miezin FM, et al. 2010. A parcellation scheme for human left lateral parietal cortex. *Neuron* 67: 156–170.

Ng L, Bernard A, Lau C, Overly CC, Dong HW, et al. 2009. An anatomic gene expression atlas of the adult mouse brain. *Nat Neurosci* 12: 356–362.

Nir Y, Mukamel R, Dinstein I, Privman E, Harel M, et al. 2008. Interhemispheric correlations of slow spontaneous neuronal fluctuations revealed in human sensory cortex. *Nat Neurosci* 11: 1100–1108.

Noble D. 2002. Modeling the heart—From genes to cells to the whole organ. *Science* 295: 1678–1682.

Norris BJ, Wenning A, Wright TM, Calabrese RL. 2011. Constancy and variability in the output of a central pattern generator. *J Neurosci* 31: 4663–4674.

Nunez PL. 2000. Towards a quantitative description of large scale neocortical dynamic behavior and EEG. *Behav Brain Sci* 23: 371–398.

Obersteiner H. 1890. *The Anatomy of the Central Nervous Organs in Health and Disease.* Philadelphia: Blakiston.

Ohiorhenuan IE, Mechler F, Purpura KP, Schmid AM, Hu Q, et al. 2010. Sparse coding and high-order correlations in fine-scale cortical networks. *Nature* 466: 617–621.

Ohki K, Reid RC. 2007. Specificity and randomness in the visual cortex. *Curr Opin Neurobiol* 17: 401–407.

Ostroff LE, Cain CK, Bedont J, Monfils MH, LeDoux JE. 2010. Fear and safety learning differentially affect synapse size and dendritic translation in the lateral amygdala. *Proc Natl Acad Sci USA* 107: 9418–9423.

Page L, Brin S, Motwani R, Winograd T. 1999. The PageRank Citation Ranking: Bringing Order to the Web. Technical Report, Stanford InfoLab.

Pakkenberg B, Pelvig D, Marner L, Bundgaard MJ, Gundersen HJ, et al. 2003. Aging and the human neocortex. *Exp Gerontol* 38: 95–99.

Palm C, Axer M, Graessel D, Dammers J, Lindemeyer J, et al. 2010. Towards ultra-high resolution fibre tract mapping of the human brain—Registration of polarized light images and reorientation of fibre vectors. *Front Hum Neurosci* 4: 9.

Pan YA, Livet J, Sanes JR, Lichtman JW, Schier AF. 2011. Multicolor Brainbow Imaging in Zebrafish. Cold Spring Harb Protoc pdb.prot5546.

Parada LA, McQueen PG, Misteli T. 2004. Tissue-specific spatial organization of genomes. *Genome Biol* 5: R44.

Parker D. 2010. Neuronal network analyses: Premises, promises and uncertainties. *Phil Trans R Soc B* 365: 2315–2328.

Passingham RE, Stephan KE, Kötter R. 2002. The anatomical basis of functional localization in the cortex. *Nat Rev Neurosci* 3: 606–616.

Pawela CP, Biswal BB, Cho YR, Kao DS, Li R, et al. 2008. Resting-state functional connectivity of the rat brain. *Magn Reson Med* 59: 1021–1029.

Pennisi E. 2000. And the gene number is ...? *Science* 288: 1146–1147.

Penny WD, Stephan KE, Mechelli A, Friston KJ. 2004. Comparing dynamic causal models. *Neuroimage* 22: 1157–1172.

Perge JA, Niven JE, Mugnaini E, Balasubramanian V, Sterling P. 2012. Why do axons differ in caliber? *J Neurosci* 32: 626–638.

Perin R, Berger TK, Markram H. 2011. A synaptic organizing principle for cortical neuronal groups. *Proc Natl Acad Sci USA* 108: 5419–5424.

Pernice V, Staude B, Cardanobile S, Rotter S. 2011. How structure determines correlations in neuronal networks. *PLoS Comput Biol* 7: e10002059.

Petreanu L, Mao T, Sternson SM, Svoboda K. 2009. The subcellular organization of neocortical excitatory connections. *Nature* 457: 1142–1145.

Phillips S, Wilson WH. 2010. Categorical compositionality: A category theory explanation for the systematicity of human cognition. *PLoS Comput Biol* 6: e1000858.

Plenz D, Thiagarajan TC. 2007. The organizing principles of neuronal avalanches: Cell assemblies in the cortex? *Trends Neurosci* 30: 101–110.

Plomin R, Haworth CMA, Davis OSP. 2009. Common disorders are quantitative traits. *Nat Rev Genet* 10: 872–878.

Poirazi P, Brannon T, Mel BW. 2003. Pyramidal neuron as two-layer neural network. *Neuron* 37: 989–999.

Poldrack RA. 2006. Can cognitive processes be inferred from neuroimaging data? *Trends Cogn Sci* 10: 59–63.

Poldrack RA, Halchenko YO, Hanson SJ. 2009. Decoding the large-scale structure of brain function by classifying mental states across individuals. *Psychol Sci* 20: 1364–1372.

Poldrack RA, Kittur A, Kalar D, Miller E, Seppa C, et al. 2011. The cognitive atlas: Toward a knowledge foundation for cognitive neuroscience. *Front Neuroinf* 5: 17.

Polsky A, Mel BW, Schiller J. 2004. Computational subunits in thin dendrites of pyramidal cells. *Nat Neurosci* 7: 621–627.

Power JD, Cohen AL, Nelson SM, Wig GS, Barnes KA, et al. 2011. Functional network organization of the human brain. *Neuron* 72: 665–678.

Price CJ, Friston JL. 2005. Functional ontologies for cognition: The systematic definition of structure and function. *Cogn Neuropsychol* 22: 262–275.

Price JC, Guan S, Burlingame A, Prusiner SB, Ghaemmaghami S. 2010. Analysis of proteome dynamics in the mouse brain. *Proc Natl Acad Sci USA* 107: 14508–14513.

Przytycka TM, Singh M, Slonim DK. 2010. Toward the dynamic interactome: It's about time. *Brief Bioinf* 11: 15–29.

Raichle ME, MacLeod AM, Snyder AZ, Powers WJ, Gusnard DA, Shulman GL. 2001. A default mode of brain function. *Proc Natl Acad Sci USA* 98: 676–682.

Raichle ME, Mintun MA. 2006. Brain work and brain imaging. *Annu Rev Neurosci* 29: 449–476.

Raichle ME. 2011. The restless brain. *Brain Connectivity* 1: 3–12.

Rajapakse I, Groudine M. 2011. On emerging nuclear order. *J Cell Biol* 192: 711–721.

Rashevsky N. 1948. *Mathematical Biophysics*. Chicago: University of Chicago Press.

Ratti C, Sobolevsky S, Calabrese F, Andris C, Reades J, et al. 2010. Redrawing the map of Great Britain from a network of human interactions. *PLoS ONE* 5: e14248.

Rein K, Zöckler M, Mader MT, Grübel C, Heisenberg M. 2002. The *Drosophila* standard brain. *Curr Biol* 12: 227–231.

Renart A, de la Rocha J, Bartho P, Hollender L, Parga N, et al. 2010. The asynchronous state in cortical circuits. *Science* 327: 587–590.

Richards EJ. 2006. Inherited epigenetic variation—Revisiting soft inheritance. *Nat Rev Genet* 5: 395–401.

Richiardi J, Eryilmaz H, Schwartz S, Vuilleumier P, Van De Ville D. 2011. Decoding brain states from fMRI connectivity graphs. *Neuroimage* 56: 616–626.

Ringo JL. 1991. Neuronal interconnection as a function of brain size. *Brain Behav Evol* 38: 1–6.

Rivera-Alba M, Vitaladevuni SN, Michchenko Y, Lu Z, Takemura S, et al. 2011. Wiring economy and volume exclusion determine neuronal placement in the *Drosophila* brain. *Curr Biol* 21: 2000–2005.

Rockel AJ, Hiorns RW, Powell TP. 1980. The basic uniformity in structure of the neocortex. *Brain* 103: 221–244.

Rockland KS. 2010. Five points on columns. *Front Neuroanat* 4: 22.

Rual JF, Venkatesan K, Hao T, et al. 2005. Towards a proteomescale map of the human protein–protein interaction network. *Nature* 437: 1173–1178.

Rubinov M, Sporns O. 2010. Complex network measures of brain connectivity: Uses and interpretations. *Neuroimage* 2: 10.

Rubinov M, Sporns O. 2011. Weight-conserving characterization of complex functional brain networks. *Neuroimage* 56: 2068–2079.

Rubinov M, Sporns O, Thivierge JP, Breakspear M. 2011. Neurobiologically realistic determinants of self-organized criticality in networks of spiking neurons. *PLoS Comput Biol* 7: e1002038.

Sandberg A, Bostrom N. 2008. *Whole Brain Emulation: A Roadmap*. Technical Report #2008–3, Future of Humanity Institute, Oxford University.

Sauer U, Heinemann M, Zamboni N. 2007. Getting closer to the whole picture. *Science* 316: 593–597.

Scannell JW, Blakemore C, Young MP. 1995. Analysis of connectivity in the cat cerebral cortex. *J Neurosci* 15: 1463–1483.

Scannell JW, Burns GAPC, Hilgetag CC, O'Neil MA, Young MP. 1999. The connectional organization of the cortico-thalamic system of the cat. *Cereb Cortex* 9: 277–299.

Schall JD. 2004. On building a bridge between brain and behavior. *Annu Rev Psychol* 55: 23–50.

Schmahmann JD, Pandya DN, Wang R, Dai G, D'Arceuil HE, et al. 2007. Association fibre pathways of the brain: Parallel observations from diffusion spectrum imaging and autoradiography. *Brain* 130: 630–653.

Schölvinck ML, Maier A, Ye FQ, Duyn JH, Leopold DA. 2010. Neural basis of global resting-state fMRI activity. *Proc Natl Acad Sci USA* 107: 10238–10243.

Scholz J, Klein MC, Behrens TEJ, Johansen-Berg H. 2009. Training induces changes in white-matter architecture. *Nat Neurosci* 12: 1370–1371.

Schwanhäusser B, Busse D, Li N, Dittmar G, Schuchhardt J, et al. 2011. Global quantification of mammalian gene expression control. *Nature* 473: 337–342.

Seung HS. 2012. *Connectome: How the Brain's Wiring Makes Us Who We Are*. New York: Houghton Mifflin Harcourt.

Shehzad Z, Kelly AM, Reiss PT, Gee DG, Gotimer K, et al. 2009. The resting brain: Unconstrained yet reliable. *Cereb Cortex* 19: 2209–2229.

Sherbondy AJ, Dougherty RF, Ananthanarayanan R, Modha DS, Wandell BA. 2009. Think global, act local: Projectome estimation with BlueMatter. *LNCS* 5761: 861–868.

Sherbondy AJ, Rowe MC, Alexander DC. 2010. MicroTrack: An algorithm for concurrent projectome and microstructure estimation. In: Jiang T et al. (eds), *LNCS 6361*, pp. 183–190. Berlin: Springer.

Shirer WR, Ryali S, Rykhlevskaia E, Menon V, Greicius MD. 2012. Decoding subject-driven cognitive states with whole-brain connectivity patterns. *Cereb Cortex* 22: 158–165.

Shmuel A, Leopold DA. 2008. Neuronal correlates of spontaneous fluctuations in fMRI signals in monkey visual cortex: Implications for functional connectivity at rest. *Hum Brain Mapp* 29: 751–761.

Sholl DA. 1956. *The Organisation of the Cerebral Cortex*. London: Methuen.

Sidaros A, Engberg AW, Sidaros K, Liptrot MG, Herning M, et al. 2008. Diffusion tensor imaging during recovery from severe traumatic brain injury and relation to clinical outcome: A longitudinal study. *Brain* 131: 559–572.

Sigrist SJ, Sabatini BL. 2012. Optical super-resolution microscopy in neurobiology. *Curr Opin Neurobiol* 22: 86–93.

Silva AJ, Zhou Y, Rogerson T, Shobe J, Balaji J. 2009. Molecular and cellular approaches to memory allocation in neural circuits. *Science* 326: 391–395.

Skudlarski P, Jagannathan K, Calhoun VD, Hampson M, Skudlarska BA, et al. 2008. Measuring brain connectivity: Diffusion tensor imaging validates resting state temporal correlations. *Neuroimage* 43: 554–561.

Skudlarski P, Jagannathan K, Anderson K, Stevens MC, Calhoun VD, et al. 2010. Brain connectivity is not only lower but different in schizophrenia: A combined anatomical and functional approach. *Biol Psychiatry* 68: 61–69.

Smith SM, Fox PT, Miller KL, Glahn DC, Fox PM, et al. 2009. Correspondence of the brain's functional architecture during activation and rest. *Proc Natl Acad Sci USA* 106: 13040–13045.

Smith SM, Miller KL, Moeller S, Xu J, Auerbach EJ et al. 2012. Temporally-independent functional modes of spontaneous brain activity. *Proc Natl Acad Sci USA* 109: 3131–3136.

Smith SM, Miller KL, Salimi-Khorshidi G, Webster M, Beckmann CF, et al. 2011. Network modeling methods for FMRI. *Neuroimage* 54: 875–891.

Song S, Sjöström PJ, Reigl M, Nelson S, Chklovskii DB. 2005. Highly nonrandom features of synaptic connectivity in local cortical circuits. *PLoS Biol* 3: e68.

Sorg C, Riedl V, Mühlau M, Calhoun V, Eichele T, et al. 2007. Selective changes of resting-state networks in individuals at risk for Alzheimer's disease. *Proc Natl Acad Sci USA* 104: 18760–18765.

Southern J, Pitt-Francis J, Whiteley J, Stokeley D, Kobashi H, et al. 2008. Multi-scale computational modelling in biology and physiology. *Prog Biophys Mol Biol* 96: 60–89.

Sporns O, Jenkinson S. 1998. Potassium ion- and nitric oxide-induced exocytosis from populations of hippocampal synapses during synaptic maturation in vitro. *Neuroscience* 80: 1057–1073.

Sporns O, Tononi G, Edelman GM. 2000. Theoretical neuroanatomy: Relating anatomical and functional connectivity in graphs and cortical connection matrices. *Cereb Cortex* 10: 127–141.

Sporns O, Chialvo D, Kaiser M, Hilgetag CC. 2004. Organization, development and function of complex brain networks. *Trends Cogn Sci* 8: 418–425.

Sporns O, Zwi J. 2004. The small world of the cerebral cortex. *Neuroinformatics* 2: 145–162.

Sporns O, Tononi G, Kötter R. 2005. The human connectome: A structural description of the human brain. *PLoS Comput Biol* 1: 245–251.

Sporns O, Honey CJ, Kötter R. 2007. Identification and classification of hubs in brain networks. *PLoS ONE* 2: e1049.

Sporns O. 2011a. *Networks of the Brain*. Cambridge: MIT Press.

Sporns O. 2011b. The non-random brain: Efficiency, economy, and complex dynamics. *Front Comput Neurosci* 5: 5.

Sporns O. 2011c. The human connectome: A complex network. *Ann N Y Acad Sci* 1224: 109–125.

Sporns O. 2012. From simple graphs to the connectome: Networks in neuroscience. *Neuroimage* doi: 10.1016/j.neuroimage.2011.08.085.

Stam CJ, Reijneveld JC. 2007. Graph theoretical analysis of complex networks in the brain. *Nonlinear Biomed Phys* 1: 3.

Stam CJ, Jones BF, Nolte G, Breakspear M, Scheltens P. 2007. Small-world networks and functional connectivity in Alzheimer's disease. *Cereb Cortex* 17: 92–99.

Stam CJ, van Straaten ECW. 2012. The organization of physiological brain networks. *Clin Neurophysiol* doi: 10.1016/j.clinph.2012.01.011.

Star EN, Kwiatkowski DJ, Murthy VN. 2002. Rapid turnover of actin in dendritic spines and its regulation by activity. *Nat Neurosci* 5: 239–246.

Stephan KE, Tittgemeyer M, Knösche TR, Moran RJ, Friston KJ. 2009. Tractography-based priors for dynamic causal models. *Neuroimage* 47: 1628–1638.

Stettler DD, Yamahachi H, Li W, Denk W, Gilbert CD. 2006. Axons and synaptic boutons are highly dynamic in adult visual cortex. *Neuron* 49: 877–887.

Stevens CF. 1989. How cortical interconnectedness varies with network size. *Neural Comput* 1: 473–479.

Stevens WD, Buckner RL, Schacter DL. 2010. Correlated low-frequency BOLD fluctuations in the resting human brain are modulated by recent experience in category-preferential visual regions. *Cereb Cortex* 20: 1997–2006.

Sugar J, Witter MP, van Strien NM, Cappaert NLM. 2011. The retrosplenial cortex: Intrinsic connectivity and connections with the (para)hippocampal regions in the rat. An interactive connectome. *Front Neuroinf* 5: 7.

Sullivan L. 1896. The tall office building artistically considered. *Lippincott's Monthly Magazine* 57: 403–409.

Supekar K, Musen M, Menon V. 2009. Development of large-scale functional brain networks in children. *PLoS Biol* 7: e1000157.

Supekar K, Uddin LQ, Prater K, Amin H, Greicius MD, et al. 2010. Development of functional and structural connectivity within the default mode network in young children. *Neuroimage* 52: 290–301.

Swanson LW. 2007. Quest for the basic plan of nervous system circuitry. *Brain Res Brain Res Rev* 55: 356–372.

Takahashi E, Dai G, Wang R, Ohki K, Rosen GD, et al. 2010. Development of cerebral fiber pathways in cats revealed by diffusion spectrum imaging. *Neuroimage* 49: 1231–1240.

Taylor AL, Goalliard JM, Marder E. 2009. How multiple conductances determine electro-physiological properties in a multicompartment model. *J Neurosci* 29: 5573–5586.

Telesford QK, Simpson SL, Burdette JH, Hayasaka S, Laurienti PJ. 2011. The brain as a complex system: Using network science as a tool for understanding the brain. *Brain Connectivity* 1: 295–308.

Thompson RH, Swanson LW. 2010. Hypothesis-driven structural connectivity analysis supports network over hierarchical model of brain architecture. *Proc Natl Acad Sci USA* 107: 15235–15239.

Thomson AM, West DC, Wang Y, Bannister AP. 2002. Synaptic connections and small circuits involving excitatory and inhibitory neurons in layers 2–5 of adult rat and cat neocortex: Triple intracellular recordings and biocytin labeling in vitro. *Cereb Cortex* 12: 936–953.

Tomasi D, Volkow ND. 2010. Functional connectivity density mapping. *Proc Natl Acad Sci USA* 107: 9885–9890.

Tomasi D, Volkow ND. 2011a. Functional connectivity hubs in the human brain. *Neuroimage* 57: 908–917.

Tomasi D, Volkow ND. 2011b. Association between functional connectivity hubs and brain networks. *Cereb Cortex* 21: 2003–2013.

Tomita M. 2001. Whole-cell simulation: A grand challenge of the 21st century. *Trends Biotechnol* 19: 205–210.

Torben-Nielsen B, Stiefel KM. 2009. Systematic mapping between dendritic function and structure. *Network* 20: 69–105.

Trachtenberg JT, Chen BE, Knott GW, Feng G, Sanes JR, et al. 2002. Long-term in vivo imaging of experience-dependent synaptic plasticity in adult cortex. *Nature* 420: 788–794.

Travers J, Milgram S. 1969. An experimental study of the small world problem. *Sociometry* 32: 425–443.

Tripodi M, Evers JF, Mauss A, Bate M, Landgraf M. 2008. Structural homeostasis: Compensatory adjustments of dendritic arbor geometry in response to variations of synaptic input. *PLoS Biol* 6: e260.

Tsuriel S, Geva R, Zamorano P, Dresbach T, Boeckers T, et al. 2006. Local sharing as a predominant determinant of synaptic matrix molecular dynamics. *PLoS Biol* 4: e271.

Tuch DS, Reese TG, Wiegell MR, Wedeen VJ. 2003. Diffusion MRI of complex neural architecture. *Neuron* 40: 885–895.

Turaga SC, Murray JF, Jain V, Roth F, Helmstaedter M, et al. 2010. Convolutional networks can learn to generate affinity graphs for image segmentation. *Neural Comput* 22: 511–538.

Tyszka JM, Kennedy DP, Adolphs R, Paul LK. 2011. Intact bilateral resting-state networks in the absence of the corpus callosum. *J Neurosci* 31: 15154–15162.

Vaishnavi SN, Vlassenko AG, Rundle MM, Snyder AZ, Mintun MA, et al. 2010. Regional aerobic glycolysis in the human brain. *Proc Natl Acad Sci USA* 107: 17757–17762.

Valdes-Sosa PA, Roebroeck A, Daunizeau J, Friston K. 2011. Effective connectivity: Influence, causality and biophysical modeling. *Neuroimage* 58: 339–361.

Van den Heuvel MP, Mandl RCW, Kahn RS, Hulshoff Pol HE. 2009a. Functionally linked resting-state networks reflect the underlying structural connectivity architecture of the human brain. *Hum Brain Mapp* 30: 3127–3141.

Van den Heuvel MP, Stam CJ, Kahn RS, Hulshoff Pol HE. 2009b. Efficiency of functional brain networks and intellectual performance. *J Neurosci* 29: 7619–7624.

Van den Heuvel MP, Hulshoff Pol HE. 2010. Exploring the brain network: A review on resting-state fMRI functional connectivity. *Eur Neuropsychopharmacol* 20: 519–534.

Van den Heuvel MP, Mandl RCW, Stam CJ, Kahn RS, Hulshoff Pol HE. 2010. Aberrant frontal and temporal complex network structure in schizophrenia: A graph theoretical analysis. *J Neurosci* 30: 15915–15926.

Van den Heuvel MP, Sporns O. 2011. Rich-club organization of the human connectome. *J Neurosci* 31: 15775–15786.

Van de Ville D, Britz J, Michel CM. 2010. EEG microstate sequences in healthy humans at rest reveal scale-free dynamics. *Proc Natl Acad Sci USA* 107: 18179–18184.

Van Dijk KRA, Hedden T, Venkataraman A, Evans KC, Lazar SW, et al. 2010. Intrinsic functional connectivity as a tool for human connectomics: Theory, properties, and optimization. *J Neurophysiol* 103: 297–321.

Van Driel R, Fransz PF, Verschure PJ. 2003. The eukaryotic genome: A system regulated at different hierarchical levels. *J Cell Sci* 116: 4067–4075.

Van Essen DC. 1997. A tension-based theory of morphogenesis and compact wiring in the central nervous system. *Nature* 385: 313–318.

Van Essen DC. 2004. Organization of visual areas in Macaque and human cerebral cortex. In: Chalupa L, Werner JS (eds), *The Visual Neurosciences*, pp. 507–521. Cambridge: MIT Press.

Van Essen DC, Ugurbil K. 2012. The future of the human connectome. *Neuroimage* doi: 10.1016/j.neuroimage.2012.01.032.

Van Gehuchten A. 1894. *Le Système Nerveux de L'Homme*. Louvain: Uystpuyst-Dieudonné.

Varkuti B, Cavusoglu M, Kullik A, Schiffler B, Veit R, et al. 2011. Quantifying the link between anatomical connectivity, gray matter volume and regional cerebral blood flow: An integrative MRI study. *PLoS ONE* 6: e14801.

Varshney LR, Chen BL, Paniagua E, Hall DH, Chklovskii DB. 2011. Structural properties of the *Caenorhabditis elegans* neuronal network. *PLoS Comput Biol* 7: e1001066.

Veraart J, Leergaard TB, Antonsen BT, Van Hecke W, Blockx I, et al. 2011. Population-averaged diffusion tensor imaging atlas of the Sprague Dawley rat brain. *Neuroimage* 58: 975–983.

Vincent JL, Patel GH, Fox MD, Snyder AZ, Baker JT, et al. 2007. Intrinsic functional architecture in the anaesthetized monkey brain. *Nature* 447: 83–86.

Vlassenko AG, Vaishnavi SN, Couture L, Sacco D, Shannon BJ, et al. 2010. Spatial correlation between aerobic glycolysis and amyloid-β (Aβ) deposition. *Proc Natl Acad Sci USA* 107: 17763–17767.

Von Bertalanffy L. 1968. *General Systems Theory*. New York: Braziller.

Voss HU, Uluc AM, Dyke JP, Watts R, Kobylarz EJ, et al. 2006. Possible axonal regrowth in late recovery from the minimally conscious state. *J Clin Invest* 116: 2005–2011.

Walker L, Chang LC, Koay CG, Sharma N, Cohen L. 2010. Effects of physiological noise in population analysis of diffusion tensor MRI data. *Neuroimage* 54: 1168–1177.

Wang J, Zuo X, He Y. 2010. Graph-based network analysis of resting-state functional MRI. *Front Syst Neurosci* 4: 16.

Wang JH, Zuo XN, Gohel S, Milham MP, Biswal BB, et al. 2011a. Graph theoretical analysis of functional brain networks: Test–retest evaluation on short- and long-term resting-state functional MRI data. *PLoS ONE* 6: e21976.

Wang Q, Gao E, Burkhalter A. 2011b. Gateways of ventral and dorsal streams in mouse visual cortex. *J Neurosci* 31: 1905–1918.

Wang Q, Sporns O, Burkhalter A. 2012. Network analysis of corticocortical connections reveals ventral and dorsal processing streams in mouse visual cortex. *J Neurosci* 32: 4386–4399.

Watson JD, Crick FHC. 1953. A structure for deoxyribose nucleic acid. *Nature* 171: 737–738.

Watson JD. 1990. The human genome project: Past, present, and future. *Science* 248: 44–49.

Watts DJ, Strogatz SH. 1998. Collective dynamics of "small-world" networks. *Nature* 393: 440–442.

Watts DJ. 2007. A twenty-first century science. *Nature* 445: 489.

Wedeen VJ, Hagmann P, Tseng WY, Reese TG, Weisskoff RM. 2005. Mapping complex tissue architecture with diffusion spectrum magnetic resonance imaging. *Magn Reson Med* 54: 1377–1386.

Wedeen VJ, Rosene DL, Wang R, Dai G, Mortazavi F, et al. 2012. The geometric structure of the brain fiber pathways. *Science* 335: 1628–1634.

Wedeen VJ, Wang RP, Schmahmann JD, Benner T, Tseng WYI, et al. 2008. Diffusion spectrum magnetic resonance imaging (DSI) tractography of crossing fibers. *Neuroimage* 41: 1267–1277.

Wedeen VJ, Wang R, Schmahmann JD, Takahashi E, Kaas JH, et al. 2009. Diffusion spectrum MRI in three mammals: Rat, monkey and human. *Front Neurosci* 3: 74–77.

Weible AP, Schwarcz L, Wickersham IR, Deblander L, Wu H, et al. 2010. Transgenic targeting of recombinant rabies virus reveals monosynaptic connectivity of specific neurons. *J Neurosci* 30: 16509–16513.

White BR, Bauer AQ, Snyder AZ, Schlaggar BL, Lee JM, et al. 2011. Imaging of functional connectivity in the mouse brain. *PLoS ONE* 6: e16322.

White JG, Southgate E, Thomson JN, Brenner S. 1983. Factors that determine connectivity in the nervous system of *Caenorhabditis elegans*. *Cold Spring Harb Symp Quant Biol* 48: 633–640.

White JG, Southgate E, Thomson JN, Brenner S. 1986. The structure of the nervous system of the nematode *Caenorhabditis elegans*. *Philos Trans R Soc Lond, B* 314: 1–340.

Wickersham IR, Finke S, Conzelmann KK, Callaway EM. 2007. Retrograde neuronal tracing with a deletion-mutant rabies virus. *Nat Methods* 4: 47–49.

Wig GS, Schlaggar BL, Petersen SE. 2011. Concepts and principles in the analysis of brain networks. *Ann N Y Acad Sci* 1224: 126–146.

Williams RW, Herrup K. 1988. The control of neuron number. *Annu Rev Neurosci* 11: 423–453.

Winkler H. 1920. *Verbreitung und Ursache der Parthenogenesis im Pflanzen- und Tierreiche.* Jena: Verlag Fischer.

Wolf L, Goldberg C, Manor N, Sharan R, Ruppin E. 2011. Gene expression in the rodent brain is associated with its regional connectivity. *PLoS Comput Biol* 7: e1002040.

Xu T, Yu X, Perlik AJ, Tobin WF, Zweig JA, et al. 2009. Rapid formation and selective stabilization of synapses for enduring motor memories. *Nature* 462: 915–919.

Yamahachi H, Marik SA, McManus JNJ, Denk W, Gilbert CD. 2009. Rapid axonal sprouting and pruning accompany functional reorganization in primary visual cortex. *Neuron* 64: 719–729.

Yang G, Pan F, Gan WB. 2009. Stably maintained dendritic spines are associated with lifelong memories. *Nature* 462: 920–924.

Yarkoni T, Poldrack RA, van Essen DC, Wager TD. 2010. Cognitive neuroscience 2.0: Building a cumulative science of human brain function. *Trends Cogn Sci* 14: 489–496.

Yarkoni T, Poldrack RA, Nichols TE, Van Essen DC, Wager TD. 2011. Large-scale automated synthesis of human functional neuroimaging data. *Nat Methods* 8: 665–670.

Yeo BTT, Krienen FM, Sepulchre J, Sabuncu MR, Lashkari D, et al. 2011. The organization of the human cerebral cortex estimated by functional connectivity. *J Neurophysiol* 106: 1125–1165.

Yook SH, Jeong HW, Barabasi AL. 2002. Modeling the Internet's large-scale topology. *Proc Natl Acad Sci USA* 99: 13382–13386.

Young MP. 1992. Objective analysis of the topological organization of the primate cortical visual system. *Nature* 358: 152–155.

Young MP. 1993. The organization of neural systems in the primate cerebral cortex. *Proc Biol Sci* 252: 13–18.

Yu JY, Kanai MI, Demir E, Jefferis GSXE, Dickson BJ. 2010. Cellular organization of the neural circuit that drives *Drosophila* courtship behavior. *Curr Biol* 20: 1602–1614.

Zalesky A, Fornito A, Bullmore ET. 2010a. Network-based statistic: Identifying differences in brain networks. *Neuroimage* 53: 1197–1207.

Zalesky A, Fornito A, Harding IH, Cocchi L, Yucel M, et al. 2010b. Whole-brain anatomical networks: Does the choice of nodes matter? *Neuroimage* 50: 970–983.

Zalesky A, Fornito A, Seal ML, Cocchi L, Westin CF, et al. 2011. Disrupted axonal fiber connectivity in schizophrenia. *Biol Psychiatry* 69: 80–89.

Zamora-López G, Zhou C, Kurths J. 2010. Cortical hubs form a module for multisensory integration on top of the hierarchy of cortical networks. *Front Neuroinf* 4: 1.

Zeki S, Shipp S. 1988. The functional logic of cortical connections. *Nature* 335: 311–317.

Zhang D, Raichle ME. 2010. Disease and the brain's dark energy. *Nature Rev Neurol* 6: 15–28.

Zhang H, Hubbard PL, Parker GJM, Alexander DC. 2011. Axon diameter mapping in the presence of orientation dispersion with diffusion MRI. *Neuroimage* 56: 1301–1315.

Zhang K, Sejnowski TJ. 2000. A universal scaling law between gray matter and white matter of the cerebral cortex. *Proc Natl Acad Sci USA* 97: 5621–5626.

Zhu X, Gerstein M, Snyder M. 2007. Getting connected: Analysis and principles of biological networks. *Genes Dev* 21: 1010–1024.

Zilles K, Amunts K. 2009. Receptor mapping: Architecture of the human cerebral cortex. *Curr Opin Neurol* 22: 331–339.

Zilles K, Amunts K. 2010. Centenary of Brodmann's map—Conception and fate. *Nat Rev Neurosci* 11: 139–145.

Zuo XN, Ehmke R, Mennes M, Imperati D, Castellanos FX, et al. 2012. Network centrality in the human functional connectome. *Cereb Cortex*.

Index